D1565140

DEMYSTIFYING STEM CELLS

DEMYSTIFYING STEM CELLS

A Real-Life Approach to Regenerative Medicine

DR. BOHDAN OLESNICKY,
DR. NAOTA HASHIMOTO, & DR. SUHYUN AN

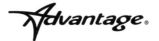

Published by Advantage, Charleston, South Carolina.
Member of Advantage Media Group.

ADVANTAGE is a registered trademark, and the Advantage colophon is a trademark of Advantage Media Group, Inc.

Printed in the United States of America.

10 9 8 7 6 5 4 3 2 1

ISBN: 978-1-64225-085-5
LCCN: 2018966789

Book design by Jamie Wise.

This publication is designed to provide accurate and authoritative information in regard to the subject matter covered. It is sold with the understanding that the publisher is not engaged in rendering legal, accounting, or other professional services. If legal advice or other expert assistance is required, the services of a competent professional person should be sought.

TreeNeutral

Advantage Media Group is proud to be a part of the Tree Neutral® program. Tree Neutral offsets the number of trees consumed in the production and printing of this book by taking proactive steps such as planting trees in direct proportion to the number of trees used to print books. To learn more about Tree Neutral, please visit **www.treeneutral.com**.

Advantage Media Group is a publisher of business, self-improvement, and professional development books and online learning. We help entrepreneurs, business leaders, and professionals share their Stories, Passion, and Knowledge to help others Learn & Grow. Do you have a manuscript or book idea that you would like us to consider for publishing? Please visit **advantagefamily.com** or call **1.866.775.1696**.

Table of Contents

A WORD FROM THE DOCTORS

Elliot B. Lander, MD, FACS, director and cofounder of Cell Surgical Network

Dr. Bohdan Olesnicky, MD

Dr. Suhyun An, DC, NP

Dr. Naota Hashimoto, DC

Who Is This Book For?

UNDERSTANDING REGENERATIVE MEDICINE

What Is Regenerative Medicine?

The Science Fiction and Science Reality of Stem Cells – Dr. Olesnicky

GETTING TO KNOW YOUR STEM CELLS

HOW DO STEM CELLS WORK?

BONE MARROW-DERIVED STEM CELLS

What Is Bone Marrow?

Bone Marrow and the Hematopoietic System

Recommendations for Sweeteners and Other Additives

Recommendations for Dairy Products

Autoimmune Conditions and the Leaky Gut

COMPLICATIONS FROM LONG-TERM DRUG USE AND CONVENTIONAL TREATMENT

Long-Term Inflammation Treatment

Non-Opioid Pain Medication and Liver Disease

Complications from General Surgery

ORTHOPEDIC PAIN

Back and Neck Pain

Knee Pain

Hip Pain

Shoulder Pain

Ankle Pain

Supportive Therapies

NEUROLOGICAL AND AUTOIMMUNE CONDITIONS

Multiple Sclerosis

Treatment of Peripheral Neuropathy

Treatment of Spinal Cord Injuries

NEW BREAKTHROUGHS IN REGENERATIVE MEDICINE THROUGH PRP

COSMETIC USES FOR REGENERATIVE MEDICINE

Mesotherapy for the Hair

Introduction

A WORD FROM THE DOCTORS

Stem cell therapy is a complicated field, and we need a diversity of opinions and insight in order to fully understand it. But most people, when they pick up a book like this, end up feeling completely overwhelmed by all of the information and technical jargon that they read. It can be a lot to take in, making it hard to read, and even harder to write. As medical professionals, we have to often remind ourselves that the public is not familiar with medical terminology.

We have to make sure that we keep our terminology generic enough to be understood by those who have not gone through four years of medical school, and, at the same time, we must provide enough detail for physicians who want to read about these procedures, or even have a procedure done. In order to get this balance right, we have approached our topic from several different angles.

There are many individuals who are eager to learn about stem cells and what they could do for their health conditions. Those suffering from knee, hip, or back pain, or some other debilitating condition, will probably browse through the introduction and then head straight to the chapter on the specific condition they are suffering from. If this is the case for you, I would highly recommend going though chapters 1 through 3 for the basics, and then chapters 7 and 9 for information on deployment and procedures.

You can then take a look at chapter 10 to learn about the dangers of leaving such conditions untreated. From here you can browse through chapters 11 and 12, where you will find more detailed information on treatment for the specific injury you may be suffering. Beyond these chapters, chapter 13 contains information on treatments utilizing growth factors. Chapter 14 is about cosmetic therapies. Chapter 15 covers therapies for sexual dysfunction. The final chapter discusses stem cell banking and how regenerative therapies can reverse the effects of aging.

This book is only intended as a guide to regenerative therapy. Your regenerative therapy specialist will let you know what method is best for your specific condition. The information presented in these pages draws on the experience and viewpoints of several medical professionals. So, before we dive into the meat and potatoes of research findings on stem cells and stem cell therapies, we should let the doctors who made this book possible introduce themselves.

ELLIOT B. LANDER, MD, FACS, DIRECTOR AND COFOUNDER OF CELL SURGICAL NETWORK

In 2010, my partner Dr. Mark Berman and I used technology brought back from Japan and South Korea to isolate high numbers of viable stem cells from small quantities of liposuction material, which, in turn, allowed us to transfer millions of healing stem cells from healthy tissue to other parts of the body that were damaged, diseased, or degenerated. We understood that this gave us an opportunity to provide our patients with regenerative cell therapy on an investigational basis under the auspices of an institutional review board (IRB) bioethics committee.

A simple, outpatient procedure gave us the opportunity to treat patients with their own stem cells—in *a completely new way*. Instead of relying on the traditional pathways, such as case studies conducted by large universities and major pharmaceutical companies that may span ten to twenty years at a time, we have greatly simplified the process.

Our stem cell procedure can be done safely and with complete sterility in the office of any physician who has the proper training and equipment. The importance of sharing information about this procedure with other physicians became clear to us early on. We wanted others to help us achieve our vision that stem cell therapy could and should be available in every doctor's office in the USA today.

We have gained wide experience and knowledge in treating thousands of patients, and we have been very fortunate to work with some of the finest physicians in America, helping them bring this regenerative technology to their practices so their patients can heal in a natural way. We have collected data indicating this procedure is safe and beneficial for a variety of medical conditions. We are very gratified to see the collaboration of high-caliber physicians such as Dr. An, Dr. Olesnicky, and Dr. Hashimoto, who are not only treating patients with our procedure but also spreading the word, providing education to the public through books such as the one you are reading right now.

You see, *Demystifying Stem Cells* was written with public service in mind. Our Cell Surgical Network's investigational stem cell technology is now used all over the world, and the core model is used by our physicians to help their patients. It is an honor to work with the very best of the best. I hope readers of this book will share with others what they learn about this exciting new stem cell revolution.

TESTIMONIALS

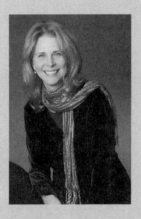

"I had stem cell therapy for the pain I was having in my hip. The procedure was relatively painless and was much more appealing than the possibility of needing surgery. The process was completed in just one day. I came into the office. They extracted some fat from my side, and prepared it to be injected into my hip. I had the remaining stem cells run through an IV for general wellness.

"Within a few months, my hip pain was significantly improved and continued to be so for several more months. I had a bit of arthritis in one of my fingers, which I wasn't really thinking about much in this procedure, yet it is completely gone. I also noticed that my skin in general was softer and moister.

"Overall, this was a good experience with very little downtime. I'm happy I did it."

Lindsay Wagner

Actor, human potential advocate

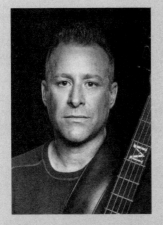

"Being a professional guitarist requires me to practice and play, on tour, at a high level, and my ability to perform at a show has a direct correlation with my ability to provide for my family. When I was younger, playing guitar in Nickelback was not a big deal at all. We would be able to practice for hours and play for days on end when we were on tour. Now that I'm starting to get a little older, I have been developing a lot of shoulder and elbow pain. Cortisone injections and surgery weren't things I wanted to pursue. That's when a friend told me about stem cell therapy. I heard about Dr. O. from some friends of mine and decided that this was something I needed to investigate. When I arrived, he performed a thorough evaluation and let me know I was a candidate. I was hopeful that this could reduce some of my chronic pain, but I was blown away at how much better I got.

"Not only was the pain gone; I was hitting chords at speeds that I hadn't done in well over a decade. Recently, we were on tour throughout Europe, and I wasn't suffering at all on the road. This treatment was a blessing, and now I don't dread the evening after a performance, because I honestly feel great.

"I haven't had to ice or take pain pills, and I honestly feel like I'm in my twenties again. I would highly recommend this to anyone because this treatment has changed my life and my ability to be a musician."

—Mike Kroeger

Musician, Nickelback

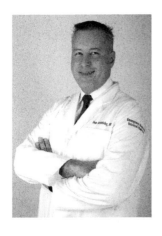

DR. BOHDAN OLESNICKY, MD

I have collaborated with Dr. Suhyun An and Dr. Naota to write an up-to-date version of *Demystifying Stem Cells: A Real-Life Approach To Regenerative Medicine.* There have been so many changes since our first book: medical advances, the discovery of new methodologies, and even the emergence of slander.

We have seen articles written by physicians stating that stem cells cannot regrow cartilage, which is 100 percent false. There are numerous scientific case studies and before-and-after images from MRIs and x-rays showing this is possible. Yet some people refuse to buy in to this therapy. Safety papers have been written, and thousands of procedures have been done without any negative incidents. Compared to surgery, this procedure is extraordinarily safe for patients.

Unfortunately, some doctors have taken a weekend seminar on our stem cell procedure and declared themselves experts on the subject. We have even seen patients who were told they were receiving stem cell therapy when, in reality, they were receiving growth factors without any stem cells at all. We wrote this book to clear up such misconceptions and have worked together to expand the original to include advances in this field and what can be offered to patients today.

Being a pioneer in this field of regenerative medicine, I have found it important to take a look at the data from different perspectives. I have worked with a wide range of health care providers with different specialties as well as different ethnic backgrounds. This is important, because our ability to view the patient and the research from different perspectives is what makes us special.

For example, I have a name that is very foreign to Americans, just as my colleagues do, but as they did, I grew up in the United States. I have a different perspective, being a second generation American. I was born and raised in New Jersey, but my parents are both physicians who lived and worked in Austria but were originally from the Ukraine. Their medical philosophy varies significantly from that of the average US physician, who believes that MD stands for "more drugs."

My parents prescribed pharmaceuticals, as I do, but I have added diet and lifestyle changes, and nutritional supplements, to my pharmaceutical interventions, and I can't tell you how many lives I have changed by doing that. Treating obese patients for lower back pain by prescribing drugs, shots, and other procedures works to some extent, but getting these patients to lose eighty pounds is what really makes the difference in their long-term outcome.

I guess this view of health seems natural to me because of my parents' influence, and over the years, I have spent some time back in the old country and have seen how medicine is practiced in other parts of the world, and I can tell you it's much different. Patients in the USA come into my office looking for a specific prescription rather than asking me to assess and recommend a treatment for them. I was enthralled with the advent of stem cell therapy because this is something I have been waiting for since the early '90s when I began researching this field.

I started stem cell research as a young man. I contemplated dropping out of medical school to pursue a career in research, but my parents insisted that I become a physician. Emergency-room (ER) medicine and internal medicine are where I got my start. I will always have a passion for ER medicine, but my true passion lies in regenerative medicine.

Treating patients with chronic neck, back, hip, knee, or shoulder pain can be extremely rewarding, especially when they have been suffering for years. We have treated patients who had surgeries that failed and who were living on pain medications. Some of them were even suicidal because of the pain. What we are offering is not just pain relief; it's a complete transformation that affects not only the patient but also everyone in their immediate family.

I can't tell you the number of people who come in to thank us because their spouse is finally getting a good night's sleep. They are so happy that their spouse is no longer a grumpy insomniac! Pain can be debilitating.

These wonderful new regenerative therapies must not be kept in the closet just because insurance companies don't yet cover them. That is why, when I have some free time, I consult with biotech firms and teach physicians about the ability of these new therapies to change patients' lives. I hope you find this book informative and will contact me or one of my colleagues if you or a loved one could benefit from these life-changing procedures.

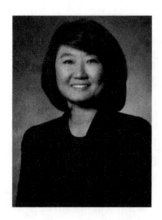

DR. SUHYUN AN, DC, NP

In my role as clinical director of the Campbell Medical Clinic, I've been treating patients for all types of chronic pain and diseases for over fifteen years, from peripheral neuropathy and multiple sclerosis to Parkinson's disease and musculoskeletal dysfunction. Sometimes I feel

I've seen it all, but in all my years of medicine, I have yet to encounter another case as dramatic as the one I witnessed with a patient named Lynn Bertrand.

When Lynn's husband wheeled her into our clinic in early 2018, it was clear the couple had nearly lost hope. Twenty years earlier, she'd been diagnosed with amyotrophic lateral sclerosis, better known as ALS or Lou Gehrig's disease, and since then her condition had gone steadily downhill. The disease had ravaged the soft muscle throughout her body, leading to a staggering array of serious issues.

Her left arm had almost completely lost all function. She'd been wheelchair bound for seventeen years. Her twenty-three-year-old son told me that he had never seen her walk on her own. And, perhaps worst of all, her weakened esophagus had caused her no end of turmoil.

"My husband has to watch as I eat," she told me, "to make sure I don't choke to death." If she lay on her back, her airway would collapse, so every night for almost twenty years, she'd been sleeping seated upright.

As with so many other patients we see, Lynn had fallen through the cracks in America's medical system. Twenty years before, a rotating cast of physicians, researchers, and other providers had poked and prodded her for months, only to ultimately confess that there wasn't much they could do for her. The only likely lasting treatment for her condition, they told her, would be stem cell therapy. But at the time, the procedure wasn't readily available in the States, and when she reached out to clinics in Europe, they quoted her an outrageous price that she couldn't afford.

Fast-forward nearly two decades, and the situation had grown dire. In response to Lynn's worsening condition, her doctors placed her in a hospice, convinced that it was only a matter of time before

ALS claimed her life. But just as the medical establishment was giving up on her, she came into Campbell Medical Clinic to attend one of our informational seminars on stem cell therapy. And with that, her life changed forever. She learned how stem cells spur the body to regenerate tissue, and how millions of patients had escaped the throes of degenerative disease with a noninvasive, safe and simple, thirty-minute treatment.

So, in a desperate final attempt to save her own life, she resolved to undergo stem cell therapy. A couple of weeks later, she came into the clinic again, this time for the procedure. And after a quick, nearly painless injection, the stem cells got to work. Two days later, I was out of the office when I received a call from a coworker who told me, "Lynn's here for her follow-up. She just strolled right in through the door with a walker!"

It was unthinkable. Lynn, who hadn't walked for nearly twenty years, was on her feet again? But after I dropped everything and rushed into the clinic to meet with her, I discovered it was all true. Lynn told me, beaming, that she was walking again. Since the treatment, she'd felt a faint but thrilling tingling sensation coursing throughout her body and had been discovering new capabilities almost constantly. Not only could she walk, but she could also eat and lie down without worry and had even regained significant use of her left arm.

Over the coming weeks, the stem cells continued their incredible work. Lynn's chronic fatigue became a thing of the past, the floaters in her eyes disappeared, and her hair even started growing back. She also felt full of youthful energy and vigor, more than she had felt in over two decades. She even started wearing makeup again. When I took her and her husband out to dinner one evening to celebrate the treatment's success, her husband watched, dumbfounded, as she ate without a care in the world.

"She never could do anything like this before," he told me with a grin. "I used to have to cut her food for her!" Six months later, she was planning a beach vacation with a few of her old friends, something she hadn't done since her diagnosis. It was beyond amazing to watch as this woman, whom I'd grown close to over the months and who had suffered so much, reclaim her ordinary, everyday life, and return to doing the things she loved to do. I felt honored to be a part of that process.

People find this story hard to believe. Skeptical doctors lecture me on how reversing the effects of ALS is impossible, let alone being able to clear up symptoms in under a week. Honestly, I get it. Lynn's transformation does indeed sound nothing short of miraculous. But the fact is *I was there*. I administered the treatment and watched as it not only allowed her to leave hospice care in the coming months but also enriched her existence in countless, meaningful ways.

What's more, while Lynn is certainly my most dramatic example of the power of stem cell therapy, she's far from the only patient who's discovered the immense benefits of the procedure. Dozens of my patients have experienced the noninvasive regenerative properties of stem cells. Rheumatoid arthritis sufferers now live without joint pain. Those afflicted by degenerative spinal disorders find themselves able to stand tall without radiating aches throughout their body. The variety of different conditions almost totally healed is huge, all thanks to these hardy little cells.

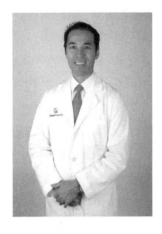

DR. NAOTA HASHIMOTO, DC

In 1999, I was involved in a head-on collision with another vehicle and suffered chronic injuries as a result of that accident. At the time, I was about to enter dental school because dentistry is what my parents thought I should be doing with the rest of my life. I had some relatives who were dentists, and who had a good relationship with my own dentist, so it was a natural career choice for me—except for the fact I wasn't passionate about it.

The precipitous event that took me off of that path was that bad car accident, which resulted in four torn ligaments—two in my cervical spine (neck), and two in my lower back and pelvis. At the time, I did everything that was asked of me by my family doctor: I took the prescribed medications and did physical therapy for about six months, with no major improvement.

I didn't like the sleepiness caused by the muscle relaxants, and the anti-inflammatories gave me stomach problems. So I was forced to suffer. When my doctor told me I needed to see an orthopedic surgeon, I panicked. After all, the last word in his title was "surgeon." Knowing what I know now, I would never have considered surgery, but try telling that to a twenty-one-year-old suffering from chronic pain. Fortunately, someone introduced me to the concept of chiropractic medicine, which eliminated all of my chronic pain issues.

The therapy combined chiropractic with physical therapy, and together with a dietary change, I was able to eliminate my pain and even cure chronic digestive and acne problems that I had suffered for years. As result of this experience, I decided to drop the idea of dental school and pursue a medical career devoted to maximizing the body's natural ability to heal itself. I used this knowledge to manage my problem for years and was even an early adopter of platelet-rich protein (PRP) therapy, with which I treated myself before it was made popular by famous athletes such as Tiger Woods.

When a colleague introduced me to Dr. Olesnicky, I found we were a natural fit. He was passionate about regenerative medicine, and I was passionate about using the body's natural ability to heal itself. We treated each other over the years. He even treated my neck, back, knee, and hair with stem cells to get my body back to tip-top shape. I shared my knowledge about dietary protocols and physical therapy with him and, over the years, we developed a great protocol for treating patients with chronic pain and other chronic conditions.

Because this is still a new field of medicine, we evaluate new research and collaborate with other doctors in the field to refine our protocols. We want to deliver the safest and most effective treatments for our patients, because if they are paying out of pocket, we cannot afford to deliver subpar results. We teamed up with Dr. An, whom we met through her work as a consultant to various allogenic facilities and umbilical cord vendors.

We all have different backgrounds, which is important because the rapid changes in this new age of medicine require us to be aware of many different perspectives. We wrote the second edition of this book because there have been many changes in techniques and regulations since the release of our 2016 edition. We hope to one day release a third edition that will account for even more changes.

WHO IS THIS BOOK FOR?

We wrote this book as a resource for those who feel they are suffering from chronic pain with no end in sight. We wrote it for anyone looking to escape persistent health problems without having to resort to the invasive, dangerous, and ineffective treatments often prescribed in our broken medical system. We're guessing that readers of this book have exhausted all other medical options.

You may be a patient whose doctor prescribed a drug with crippling side effects, or who suggested cortisone shots or another steroid. Instead of addressing the problem at the source, your doctor just threw on a band-aid, temporarily and ineffectually masking your symptoms. Perhaps another physician even recommended surgery. Despite all their initial reassurance that going under the knife would work, followed by a dangerous procedure and a lengthy rehabilitation process, you still find yourself struggling with chronic pain and disease every single day. You're fed up with this crazy merry-go-round where treatment after invasive treatment fails, while your condition steadily worsens. We can't tell you the number of patients who come into our clinics and report that they've been dealing with an issue for ten, twenty, or even thirty years without a single ounce of lasting relief. These patients' pain and struggle go far beyond mere annoyance. They're unable to sleep well at night, they can't pick up their grandchildren, and they can no longer go golfing with their buddies on the weekends.

They've worked hard their entire lives, looking forward to traveling the world during their retirement, only to find their back pain prevents them from getting on a plane. They can barely walk, cook, or even shop for their own groceries. Independence is a distant memory, replaced by constant suffering that diminishes every aspect of their well-being. They give up hope that anybody will be able to help and accept their poor health as something they have to deal with for the rest of their lives.

If any of this sounds familiar, you've come to the right place. We wrote this book for all of you out there who have restructured your day-to-day living to accommodate your disease, who have made lifestyle changes, tried countless medications, injections, and maybe even surgery, and experienced only fleeting relief at best. We also wrote this book for those afflicted by illnesses for which modern medicine has no answer, such as autoimmune diseases, rheumatoid arthritis, multiple sclerosis, fibromyalgia, and Parkinson's disease.

You don't have to suffer in silence any longer. The future of medicine is here, and it's called regenerative medicine. Throughout this book, we'll answer all your burning questions about this innovative, incredibly powerful new treatment, and we'll help you determine whether stem cell therapy is right for you. You'll discover what stem cells are, how they work, and all the amazing ways they can transform your life from the inside-out.

Despite all of the good information out there, however, there are still a lot of bad actors in the field of medicine who, after taking a weekend seminar, presume they are an expert. It is the yarns these half-baked promoters spin that have left many of you skeptical. I understand that. And it is for this reason that we wrote this book. We are determined to eliminate the confusion and completely demystify stem cells.

Chapter 1

UNDERSTANDING REGENERATIVE MEDICINE

Before doing anything else, we will go over such fundamental things as how stem cells are produced and used in regenerative medicine. So, let's get started!

WHAT IS REGENERATIVE MEDICINE?

If you sprained an ankle, skinned your knees, or had a common cold, you were a full beneficiary of the human body's unique and powerful regenerative powers. We are able to regenerate vital cells and tissues on a daily basis. This is standard procedure for all living creatures. The problem is that the potency of our own natural ability to regenerate declines with time. So, what then is regenerative medicine?

Regenerative medicine is simply a means to stoke the flames of those natural fires of human healing. Whether it is done through healing stem cell therapies, or through platelet-rich blood, regenerative medicine is aimed at restoring the body's own capacity to heal. In this book, we will take you through every nook and cranny of regenerative medicine: its history, current procedures, and future developments.

Follow along with us as we explore such captivating trends as the vampire face lift, PRP shots, and cutting-edge techniques of stem cell therapy. Regenerative medicine has no limits. When other doors of healing and recovery have closed, regenerative medicine provides us a way. We only have one life to live, so we might as well live it to its fullest. And regenerative medicine provides us with the means to do just that.

THE SCIENCE FICTION AND SCIENCE REALITY OF STEM CELLS - DR. OLESNICKY

I was recently watching an episode of *Doctor Who*, the British sci-fi show. In this episode, they used miraculous microscopic robots programmed to repair and grow tissue perfectly matched to the patient's body, based on the DNA. I laughed, not because it was science fiction, or because the screenwriter had written anything particularly funny, but because repair robots are exactly what we already have in our body in the form of stem cells. And we're using stem cells today to do things that probably would have seemed like science fiction just a few years ago.

When it comes to the successful use of stem cells, the key is figuring out where to get them from and how to make them do what we want them to do. People have been harvesting and moving tissue to different parts of the body for many years now. We're finally able to harvest these tiny little biological robots and move them to areas where we can use them instead of just storing them without benefit. We are on the cutting edge of the most incredible advance in medical technology that harnesses a blend of genetics, regenerative medicine, and Mother Nature.

Stem cells seem to be the medical buzz word of late, and for good reason. This treatment isn't just for celebrities and professional athletes anymore. Not too long ago, people who could afford to do so would travel to Germany, Russia, and Mexico to receive experimental treatments and even some treatments that are still currently banned in the USA, such as those using fetal stem cells from aborted fetuses.

One of the general public's biggest misunderstandings about stem cells comes from the use of fetal stem cells. I'd like to point out that fetuses and babies are not killed in order to harvest stem cells for medical use. However, moral and personal beliefs should no longer be an issue, because there are plenty of other types of stem cells that work just as well as, if not better than, fetal stem cells. In any event, this book is about *nonembryonic* stem cell transplantation, so read on.

Aside from the embryonic stem cell issue, it's hard for someone who is not a medical professional to filter through the plethora of information about stem cells that comes from the media, scientific journals, and the Internet. You may also wonder about the different types of regenerative procedures, such as platelet-rich protein (PRP) therapy and amniotic fluid therapy, and why the price varies. The goal of this book is to provide you with basic information about each option, and why you might choose one over the other for specific conditions.

Once you have that data, you should be able to make a decision that is right for you. We believe that stem cell transplantation is the real future of regenerative medicine. It's hard to be a skeptic when you have seen countless miracles unfold right before your eyes. The problem that most physicians have with the new field of stem cell transplantation is that they are unfamiliar with it. It wasn't taught in medical school and most physicians don't have large pharmaceutical companies behind them, funding study after study.

The reason why many private companies haven't been performing study after study is that studies cost millions of dollars. I have personal knowledge of this since I assisted in such studies in graduate school and saw their cost first-hand. In fact, I am currently working on getting a basic rubber tourniquet device through the FDA approval process. The device will cost millions of dollars just to make it available to the public.

Large companies invest millions of dollars of capital to make a medication or device publicly accessible because they will most likely be able to hold the patent for about twenty years. This means no one else can make the same product for that period of time. A successful device or medication can make a company millions, and possibly billions, of dollars during that twenty-year time span. For example, Lipitor, a cholesterol medication made by Pfizer, grossed $12.9 billion during its peak in 2006 and has grossed multiple billions every year since.

Those numbers may seem large, but if you take into consideration some of the new antibody medications, which can cost insurance companies upward of $440,000 a year, you can begin to follow the money trail. It is such funding that allows pharmaceutical companies to render tremendous profit margins, which leads to the publication of more studies, more advertising, and more lobbying to spread the word about the company's medications.

Obviously, Lipitor was a grand slam for Pfizer and others like Pfizer. Not all patents can make money like this. But profit is the reason why companies risk everything and invest millions in studies to get a device or medication to the public. To obtain a patent, you need to manufacture something that is 100 percent reproducible, and it cannot be a natural product. For example, no one gets to patent air and water and then charge for its use. Therefore, stem cells are difficult to patent because they are natural. Just how do you patent something that naturally grows in the human body?

The FDA would have to define birth tissues, bone marrow, or fat as a drug, which would then be regulated by that agency. Only then could a process be patented. Only then would you have larger companies buying up the rights to the process so they could fund studies and bring the end product to market. I'm not saying that this would be impossible, but it would definitely drive the cost much higher than it is today. In the meantime, studies are being funded to ascertain the validity of smaller clinical trials, and eventually, as more and more trials are carried out and the results published, various end products processes will become available to the public.

Unfortunately, without billions of dollars of funding, the process of clinical trials and published results will be slow. Although lack of funding can make stem cell research and the creation of stem cell therapies seem like an uphill battle, stem cell regenerative medicine is steadily marching out of the realm of science fiction and into science reality.

Chapter 2

GETTING TO KNOW YOUR STEM CELLS

While stem cells are an intrinsic part of all of us, most know very little about them. A stem cell is how we all started in life. We each had twenty-three chromosomes donated by Mom and three by Dad, and they became the stem cell that, eventually, grew into each of us. From this one tiny cell, all of our body parts, organs, and tissues develop. Pretty amazing, huh? And that is precisely why there is such a buzz about stem cell therapy.

Stem cells are immature, generative cells that have the ability to develop into a wide variety of other cells, which allows them to regenerate muscle cells, bone cells, cartilage cells, and brain cells, among others. Stem cells are a vital driver of human embryonic development and, as you age, are a primary force behind your body's ability to replenish and repair dying and damaged tissue.

The human body is comprised of many organs and tissues, all of which function as a cohesive unit to allow the body and each of its many components to properly work together. The fundamental biological unit within the body is the cell. There are many different types of cells found in various tissues throughout the body. Many of them have unique properties designed to carry out a range of specific functions.

Some cells, however, are not differentiated; they don't have specialized functions. These are our stem cells, and they, too, undergo maturation and can form more of their own kind. Stem cells consist of growth factors in, essentially, a blank template: no specialization has yet taken place, but they have the ability to be transformed into various specific cell types. Stem cell research has a long and rich history, branching into various medicinal applications for humans, as well as animals.

The terminology of stem cells was coined between the 1860s and the 1880s. German biologist Ernst Haeckel was the first to do this in 1868, before William Sedgwick followed suit nearly two decades later, in 1886. A decade and a half after stem cell terminology was first developed, scientists began to work tirelessly to uncover the secrets hidden behind these incredibly versatile cells.

It has long been known that their potential use greatly outweighs their current status as useful tools in medicine and science. At the moment, we use a wide variety of adult stem cells in our practice. They may be derived from birth tissue (amnion, placenta, or umbilical cord), or bone marrow or adipose tissue. They are taken from a patient's own body (autologous) or donated, and they are nonembryonic.

In the past, embryonic stem cells have been hailed by the media for their pluripotent property, which means they can turn into any type of cell. They originate at the embryonic development stage, where they have the ability to generate any tissue in the body, unlike adult stem cells, which are multipotent. However, studies are beginning to show that adult stem cells from areas such as bone marrow and birth tissue (placental and umbilical cord) may be better suited for adult treatment because there is no risk of forming teratomas (a type of cancerous growth).

Embryonic cells are designed to grow a human being and have an extremely rapid growth process that has great potential but also carries risk. Adult stem cells are *not* pluripotent; they are multipotent, meaning that they can develop into many different types of cells, such as those found in bone, various tissues, and fat. Most have the ability to differentiate and heal damaged tissue. You can rest assured that this type of stem cell carries a wide range of beneficial applications for regenerative medicine involving very low risk.

We can fully assure you that stem cells are the future of health care. Once activated, they can turn into any other type of cell and replicate over and over again until the damaged tissue is repaired. Stem cells perform these actions following signals from growth factors within the damaged tissue. The form of stem cell most people think of is the embryonic stem cell found in a fetus, but stem cells can be found throughout an adult body as well as in special pockets of tissue called stem cell niches.

And the type of stem cell that most practices are using is an adult mesenchymal stem cell (MSC), so-called because it comes from the mesodermal layer of a partially developed embryo. These stem cells are multipotent and are very valuable when it comes to the repair of bones, cartilage, and other connective tissue. When they are autologously derived (i.e., they come from the patient's own body), there is no risk of a patient's body rejecting them. Embryonic stem cells, on the other hand, are even more versatile than MSCs, but their use carries slightly more risk and the perception of moral baggage.

Just remember, embryonic stem cells can turn into any type of tissue in the body since the human body originated from that type of cell. Without that ability, we wouldn't be here today. But because they are gathered from aborted fetuses, some oppose their use on philosophical and moral grounds. The overall safety of using embryonic cells is high, but there is a small chance that embryonic cells could turn into cancerous tumor cells because of their rapid growth. Moreover, because embryonic tissue is not from the patient's own body, its use in the patient could lead to unforeseen problems.

Adult MSCs can turn into most types of tissue in the body and are much safer to use than embryonic stem cells. Also, ethical issues do not apply to MSCs (also called adult stem cells—ASC). They can form bone, cartilage, muscle, nerves, blood vessels, connective tissue, and fat.

That is why ASCs from the mesodermal layer work extremely well for most medical conditions. They have the ability to develop into any of the above-mentioned tissues. We will discuss this in further detail a little later in this book, but for right now, just consider the power of a simple medical procedure that could make knee-replacement surgery unnecessary by simply regrowing the knee's lost cartilage. See the tissue model below of ASCs turning into other types of cell.

Chapter 3

HOW DO STEM CELLS WORK?

In the past, those who used stem cell therapy could only theorize on how they functioned. Researchers could document the results of their studies but were not entirely clear as to how those results came about. They discovered that stem cells injected into a rat had an immediate effect, but they were not sure how those effects were produced. But with the development of newer technologies such as MRI, PET, and SPECT imaging with radionuclear tracers, scientists were able to finally measure the mysterious activity taking place within the stem cell.

These imaging studies clearly show that the stem cell and progenitor cells (stem cell descendants) are, eventually, drawn to the site of tissue injury, even if the regenerative cells were delivered by intravenous (IV) therapy. Stem cells are able to find these damaged areas because these areas release cytokine signals that will draw in stem cells and other types of healing cells to help repair the damaged cells.

Cytokines are signaling proteins that send homing beacons (instructions), to incoming cells and proteins. Bound to receptors, they are among a number of substances secreted by stem cells (and other parts of the body) that send the signals activating and recruiting stem cells for a particular job.

Where there is no injury to automatically draw the regenerative cells to the site—during an aesthetic procedure, for example—a microtrauma is created in the area to draw those regenerative cells there. Throughout this book we will discuss specific examples of some of the common procedures that clinics such as ours perform around the country. You will hear of such things as the vampire face lift, the O-Shot, and the P-Shot—all designed to restore and rejuvenate deteriorating tissue.

Once the stem cells have been activated, they need raw materials in order to do the rebuilding they've been recruited to do. That's where growth factors come in. They comprise the wide variety of compounds—for example, enzymes, electrolytes, carbohydrates, and osteogenic cofactors—that form the building blocks of biological growth. Imagine spraining your ankle. After the injury, your body's cytokines rush over to the damaged area and call in stem cells and other important healing mechanisms in your body: "Hey! Come over here and get to work!"

The stem cells make their way over to the injury and use the store of growth factors as their materials to start the reconstruction and regeneration process. It's a remarkable process with powerful results. The reason why stem cells work and achieve such dramatic results while still being completely safe for patients to use is due to the three unique properties they all share. These three properties come together to make the process as painless and seamless as possible.

These properties are the following:

First, stem cells are both antimicrobial and antiviral, clearing out dangerous bacteria and viruses through their secretion of certain types of peptides, proteins, and other compounds.

Second, they're immunomodulating, which is a fancy way of saying they can regulate and rebalance an overactive or underactive immune system. For instance, if a patient is suffering from an auto-immune disease such as rheumatoid arthritis, in which the body mistakenly attacks its own tissues, stem cells can help calm it down and drastically reduce the damage. Across the country, millions of people suffering from autoimmune diseases, including diabetes, multiple sclerosis, celiac disease, among numerous others, could benefit immensely from this process.

Third, stem cells are immunoprivileged. This means that that the immune system will not attack stem cells when they are introduced to the body.

You may be wondering how stem cells can be integrated into a patient's own immune system if they are harvested from another person, as is the case with umbilical cord blood. Do they need to be the same blood type? Is there a chance the patient's body will reject these foreign cells? But you'll remember from our discussion in the previous chapter that stem cells are immature cells. This means that they haven't had yet formed any kind of surface antigens or killer T-cells, which help the body filter out unwanted pathogens.

Because of this, nearly anyone can safely receive stem cell injections with no risk of rejection or complication. As a result, stem cell therapy is a safe, powerful procedure. And the current process that we advocate uses adult MSCs that are procured from bone marrow or fat tissue, or are purchased allogenic cells from birth tissues such as umbilical cord blood.

All of these are minor procedures with no downtime, compared to alternatives such as surgery. Stem cells are highly effective in the sense that they know their job: they immediately arrive at the scene of injury and get to work safely repairing the damaged tissue. This is how stem cells work. So now that you know how stem cells work, keep reading further to find out just how these industrious stem cell dynamos can work for you.

Chapter 4

BONE MARROW-DERIVED STEM CELLS

Bone marrow stem cells are here to stay. These stem cells have been used by doctors all around the country and have the most studies associated with them. In this chapter we will take a closer look at all the many ways these valuable cellular resources have come to benefit our lives.

WHAT IS BONE MARROW?

Bone marrow is a soft material—often referred to as spongy material—that is found in the medullary cavities of our bones. The medullary cavities are, basically, large, centralized, hollowed out shafts that serve as repositories for bone marrow. In these cavities, there are two kinds of bone marrow: red bone marrow (also called myeloid tissue), and yellow bone marrow (sometimes referred to as fatty tissue).

CHARACTERISTICS OF RED BONE MARROW

This is a very delicate structure composed of blood-forming hematopoietic stem cells.

The red color can be attributed to the high hemoglobin, an iron-rich protein responsible for carrying oxygen throughout the body.

All of our blood platelets, RBCs (red blood cells), as well as most of our WBCs (white blood cells), are produced from red bone marrow.

CHARACTERISTICS OF YELLOW BONE MARROW:

Found in the medullary cavities of long bones, yellow marrow is, typically, encased underneath a layer of red bone marrow.

- It is yellow due to a high concentration of adipose (fat) cells.
- It contains MSCs capable of producing bone, cartilage, and fat.
- Yellow marrow also produces a low level of white blood cells.
- Yellow bone marrow works as an insulator providing the proper cushioning and conditions for our bones.

Bone marrow first forms during the end of a fetus's tenure in the womb and is fully active at birth. Initially, bone marrow is primarily red, but by the time a child reaches eight years of age, much of the red marrow has been replaced by yellow marrow, and by adulthood, approximately half of the bone marrow is yellow. Bone marrow has proven itself to be a hidden resource of health in the form of stem cells.

Bone marrow stem cells are capable of healing damaged tissue and rebooting whole immune systems. But how exactly did this discovery come about? This field has had a long and fascinating history. Read further to discover the incredible origin of these cellular wonder workers.

TIMELINE OF IMPORTANT MILESTONES IN BONE MARROW RESEARCH

- Early 1900s: Bone marrow is first extracted from live patients.

- Late 1920s: Sternal aspiration of bone marrow is first introduced.

- 1956: First successful bone marrow transplant takes place.

- 1958: Yugoslavian engineers exposed to radiation from the meltdown of a nuclear reactor are given bone marrow transplants. Afterward, the first documented case of graft versus host disease was observed in the patients.

- 1960: Two types of stem cells in bone marrow are discovered: hematopoietic and MSCs.

- Early 1980s: Patients are approved for autologous bone marrow transplantation.

- 1988: Bone Marrow Donors Worldwide is established.

- 2007: Donors in the Bone Marrow Donors Worldwide database surpass eleven million.

BONE MARROW AND THE HEMATOPOIETIC SYSTEM

Bone marrow is part of what is called the hematopoietic system. It is from this system that new blood cells are formed. Many are not aware that the blood running through our veins is manufactured in our bones. The prodigious little manufacturers of this blood supply are the hematopoietic stem cells produced in our bone marrow. It is in the bone marrow that these stem cells produce red blood cells for the conveyance of oxygen, and platelets for clotting, as well as white blood cells, whose job is to bolster the immune system.

CHARACTERISTICS OF HEMATOPOIETIC STEM CELLS

- Hematopoietic stem cells are multipotent: they are able to produce a variety of blood-based materials such as blood platelets and red and white blood cells.
- They are commonly found in bone marrow but are also available in peripheral blood of the body and in umbilical cord blood.
- Hematopoietic stem cells are capable of restoring damaged and weakened immune systems.

Another type of stem cell that is found in the bone marrow of the human body is the marrow stromal stem cell (also know as a mesenchymal cell—MSC). Bone marrow-derived MSCs are able to produce several kinds of skeletal and connective tissues such as cartilage, bone, and fat. There is much in the way of promising research when it comes to the potential of bone marrow-derived MSCs to repair cartilage and bone-based diseases. These stem cells can be harvested from either the hip of the donor, or from the knee.

CHARACTERISTICS OF MSCS

- MSCs can be found in the various parts of the body but have large deposits in yellow bone marrow.
- They are multipotent and have the potential to create liver cells.
- In treatment, bone marrow MSCs are usually extracted from the knee or hip.

Hematopoietic stem cells and MSCs can also be derived from peripheral blood sources and umbilical cord blood. Currently, several cord banks across the United States specialize in the collection, processing, and storage of umbilical cord blood, which can, in turn, be used at a later date for their hematopoietic stem cells.

WHAT CAN IT BE USED FOR?

Cancer patients subjected to radiation and chemotherapy are often given bone marrow transplants in order to offset the collateral damage they have suffered as a result of their treatment. Radiation and chemo are used, of course, to destroy cancer cells, but they also destroy many healthy cells. Bone marrow transplants, however, have been found to help restore these depleted systems of the body, and of all the many stem cell therapy clinical trials currently underway at the moment, bone marrow transplant trials also have the longest standing history compared to newer types of stem cell therapy.

Besides bone marrow transplants, however, several new methodologies to treat degenerative diseases are being developed using bone marrow-derived stem cells. Some of these methods are still in their most preliminary stages of development while others are much further along. Here is an overview of some of the most prominent research currently being conducted.

EXPLORATORY THERAPIES USING BONE MARROW-DERIVED STEM CELLS

- Myocardial infarction: Several studies have shown bone marrow-based stem cells to be well dispositioned for the treatment of myocardial infarction. These stem cells seem to be highly effective in correcting ailments of the heart. Recent research efforts have documented this fact through trial runs with laboratory animals such as pigs, providing promising results. Although still in the preliminary stages, this same type of stem cell treatment, it is believed, could be used some day in the future to successfully treat heart disease patients.

- Traumatic brain injury: Another arena in which there has been much recent talk of the potential use of bone marrow-derived stem cell therapy is traumatic brain injury (TBI). As it turns out,

MSCs derived from bone marrow have quite a knack for reducing the swelling that characterizes so many traumatic brain injuries. MSCs come from natural immunosuppressive agents that can help contain and reduce swelling of the brain, thereby preventing further progression of TBI-related brain disease. MSCs are also uniquely outfitted with the ability to produce beneficial growth factors that coax the brain into rebuilding damaged neurons.

- Diabetes: It's become nothing short of a modern epidemic, and does not appear to be going away anytime soon. Treatment with bone marrow-derived stem cells holds some promise, however. Several studies have shown that when diabetic mice in the laboratory are injected with these stem cells, the incidence of their diabetes is decreased. It has been found that the stem cells, once introduced to the blood stream, go directly to the mouse's pancreas, prompting the damaged organ to repair itself. As a result of this intervention, the previously diabetic mice were able to bring both their blood sugar and their insulin levels under control. The procedure still needs more testing, but if the results continue to hold up to scrutiny, this is a diabetic treatment that many human subjects will be eager to try.

As you can see, bone marrow-derived stem cells have revolutionized the field of regenerative medicine, and the full benefits that can be gleaned from bone marrow stem cell therapy have only just begun. We will all just have to stay tuned for further developments.

HOW THE BONE MARROW PROCEDURE IS CURRENTLY BEING DONE

Bone marrow is a number-one site of stem cell extraction, but just how is extraction done? In this chapter, we will clear up any confusion about the procedures for extracting bone marrow and processing those precious stem cells locked inside. As mentioned earlier, the practice of transplanting bone marrow into a patient to encourage the production of bone marrow stem cells has existed since the 1980s.

In order to procure these stem cells, a procedure called a bone marrow biopsy is carried out. It involves the insertion of a specialized needle directly into the bone marrow to collect the stem cells. The collection site is usually the hip bone, although, in younger people, it may be possible to collect bone marrow from the sternum and upper tibia bone.

Bone marrow can be gleaned through either autologous or allogenic extraction. As mentioned earlier, autologous transplants use the patient's own bone marrow, whereas allogenic transplants involve the participation of a donor. Autologous transplants are usually preferred since the use of a patient's own tissue negates the incidence of rejection. Allogenic donations, on the other hand, may have to be coupled with strong immunosuppressive drugs to prevent rejection by the receiving patient's immune system.

The process of collecting bone marrow would be an extremely painful one without anesthesia. And since this is, obviously, a very serious procedure, the patient is, at the very least, given local anesthesia. The hip area targeted for extraction is sanitized and numbed prior to the surgical procedure. With the donor/patient properly anesthetized, the attending physician will use guided imagery to drill right into the extraction site and harvest the bone marrow stem cells. Just keep in mind that this is not as painful as a bone marrow biopsy, which some patients may have been subjected to if they had previously served as donors of bone marrow.

The harvested stem cells are processed into bone marrow aspiration concentrate (BMAC) and mixed with natural growth factors to form a special soup. This material will then be reinjected into joints, tissues, or other areas, depending on the patient's condition.

The biggest drawback to gathering stem cells from bone marrow has to do with their age. The stem cells that can be gathered from bone marrow have a somewhat limited shelf life, becoming less effective with age. This is why bone marrow transplants are so highly effective in young leukemia patients, for example, and less effective in older patients.

WHAT IS RECOVERY LIKE FOR THE PATIENT?

In reality, the downtime of this procedure is minimal. Most patients will be able to drive themselves to and from the doctor's office without any difficulty. The procedure is much less taxing than surgery and nothing compared to the excruciatingly painful bone marrow transplant you may have read about on the Internet, because far less bone marrow is extracted.

Chapter 5

ADIPOSE-DERIVED STEM CELLS

Adipose tissue is a kind of connective tissue that primarily consists of fat cells called adipocytes. As well as storing fat, adipose tissue also contains many important blood vessels and nerve cells. Adipose tissue is quite prolific and is deposited throughout most of the body. It serves as a cushion around muscles, and as insulation for internal organs. It can also be found just under the skin in the form of subcutaneous fat and is even locked inside bone marrow.

WHAT PURPOSE DOES ADIPOSE TISSUE SERVE?

Adipose tissue is a number-one source of energy for our body, so much so that many of us often store large fat deposits of it for later use. Yes, as much as we don't like it, that extra lining of fat cells around our waistline serves a purpose: our body can burn up this fat for extra energy. Of course, most of us are not too keen on lugging around big bellies of adipose-tissue energy stores!

Besides being a source of stored-up energy, adipose tissue also plays an important role in the regulation of hormones and metabolism. Adipose tissue sends messages from cell to cell in the body. Yes, it is true: fat can communicate. Recent studies have discovered that microribonucleic acids (RNAs) are used by adipose tissue to help control protein production and gene expression.

RESEARCH INTO ADIPOSE TISSUE

A technique for extracting individual adipose cells from rats was first developed in the 1960s. This technique was further refined for human application by the 1980s. Official research into the potential benefit of adipose-derived stem cells was first conducted in 1992. During this preliminary research, it was discovered that "porcine preperitoneal fat is nearly identical to human subcutaneous adipose cells in its composition. It is this this tissue that has proved to be a goldmine for multipotent stem cells." The first procedure performed in the USA was done in 2010 and utilized a technology that was derived from Asia.

Adipose tissue-derived stem cells (ADSCs), and more specifically stromal vascular fraction (SVF), have proven pivotal in the ongoing research for stem-cell-based regenerative therapy. Adipose tissue-derived stem cells have successfully regenerated everything from neural and vascular cells to osteocytes, hepatocytes, and cells and tissue of the pancreas. ADSCs are coupled with a large dose of immunosuppressive trophic factors, which ensures a very low chance of rejection among recipients. More research still needs to be done, but the results are promising.

SVF also contains macrophages, regulatory T cells, endothelial cells, red blood cells, growth factors, and micelles. The adult adipose-derived stem cells remain dormant until the occurrence of tissue injury, when they receive signals from growth factors to transform them into functioning stem cells. Fat contains five hundred thousand to 1.4 million stem/progenitor cells per milliliter, and since plenty of fat is available (at least we can find a silver lining in that storm cloud!), there are usually plenty of stem cells that can be recruited to heal the body.

Note that progenitor cells have many stem-cell qualities but cannot replicate as often or differentiate into as many types of cells as stem cells can. While they descend from stem cells, they can only differentiate into certain types of cell. Fat is made up of adipocytes and preadipocytes. Preadipocytes can multiply into additional fat cells (adipocytes) when challenged by an increase in caloric intake. Believe it or not, this is a survival mechanism, no matter how unsightly it may make one look.

If your weight remains stable, these preadipocytes will remain dormant until a fat cell dies. Then they activate and turn into new fat cells. When separated from fat and collagen, they are identical to MSCs, which is why scientists and physicians are so excited with this very recent discovery.

WHAT IS THE PROCESS FOR ADIPOSE-DERIVED STEM CELL TREATMENT?

We always use a closed, sterile surgical system for SVF production. This means that the cells are not exposed to the environment prior to deployment into the body. This virtually eliminates the chance of contamination, which, of course, is very good news to patients who can come into the office for a quick, painless procedure without any fear of cross-contamination.

Standard preoperative protocols are, of course, necessary prior to the procedure, just as they would be for any minor surgery, and include having patients report any infections, surgeries, and dental work done at least one month prior to the procedure. Patients may be required to take antibiotics if they experienced such medical conditions within that one-month window. There is no direct, mandatory restriction on the use of anti-inflammatories before or after the procedure, but some doctors might suggest the patient temporarily discontinue their use.

They may suggest the patient stops using such drugs after the procedure in order to maximize the cytokine and natural inflammatory response from the sites of injury.

The patient will be expected to take a conventional shower prior to the procedure and wash all areas thoroughly. The patient will also be expected to wear loose, comfortable clothing that can easily fit over a surgical wrap. There are no mandatory dietary restrictions before or after the procedure. However, alcohol should not be consumed within eight hours of the procedure. We also suggest that patients have only a light last meal before the procedure just in case they become nervous.

The area of fat typically used is in the posterior flank, or love handle, because of its ease of access, vascularity, and the fact there are no major organs in that area and no risk of a hernia. In extremely thin patients, we can usually find some fat near the buttocks as well. The amount of adipose fat tissue that is used to treat two to three selected areas is, typically, 50 cubic centimeters (cc) or 1.7 ounces, which is not very much at all.

In fact, many patients even suggest that while we have them locally anesthetized, we pull out much more than that! Many patients readily tell us that they have more fat that they would like to donate, but this is just a kind of running joke we go through with a lot of our patients. And no matter how much some would like to "take a little extra" around the edges, 50 cc is usually as far as we go.

Below is an illustration of the procedure. As you can see, the incision is so small you barely even notice it.

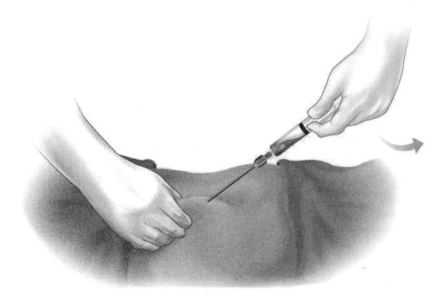

Immediately afterward, this area is cleaned up, sterilized again, and covered with a dressing to absorb any leakage of bodily fluids and blood. Finally, a piece of rubber foam is placed where the fat was harvested and a compression dressing is put on for one to two days to help smooth out the fat. Then the process of isolating the stem cells begins. This part is very technical but does not take long. After ninety minutes of work, we will have the finished product, which will be approximately 10 cc of SVF, an accumulation of fatty, yellow adipose tissue sometimes referred to as liquid gold.

Each cubic centimeter of this SVF contains between five hundred thousand and 1.4 million stem cells, which means there are between five and fourteen million stem cells per 10 cc of SVF. Once you have this liquid gold, you can either inject it into the affected area of the body and/or use IV deployment. We usually apply both since most of our patients have multiple problems.

The most wonderful characteristic of adipose-derived stem cells is that no matter what the injury may be, they automatically work to restore damaged tissue. Even after IV deployment, these cells, once introduced into the body immediately navigate to the trouble spots where they are needed. Call it liquid gold, or call it just plain fat, adipose tissue really knows how to stay on task!

Chapter 6

ALLOGENIC REGENERATIVE THERAPY: WHAT IS IT, AND WHY DOES IT MATTER? DR. AN'S REPORT

The medical use of umbilical cord tissues is far from new. For decades, we've been well aware of the immense density of powerful compounds found in the placenta and umbilical cord and have taken advantage of their unique properties to treat all kinds of issues. I've met several nurses who, back in the day, sometimes slapped human placentas over burn wounds to speed up the recovery process.

While the medical establishment definitely doesn't do this anymore, I'm passionate about the use of umbilical cord stem cells for the treatment of all kinds of disease and disorder. Over the past few years, they've enabled me to help hundreds of patients escape from chronic pain and return to doing the things they love to do.

And, perhaps best of all, the umbilical cord stem cells are sourced ethically during the natural birthing process.

THE COLLECTION PROCESS OF UMBILICAL CORD STEM CELLS

After a healthy baby is born, all the extra stuff—the umbilical cord, the placenta, the amniotic membrane and fluid—is usually considered nothing more than the waste product of the birthing process and is thrown away. But these tissues are extremely rich in those multipotent stem cells we discussed earlier—the type that is instrumental in treating chronic pain and disease. So, with the consent of the parents, these tissues can be donated to labs that bank them for later use.

Such labs go through an extensive screening and inspection process by the American Association of Tissue Banks (AATB) before they're allowed to legally harvest umbilical cord tissue. The mothers must undergo a comprehensive health screening and blood test to ensure they are not carriers of any diseases or pathogens. Then, after the baby is born, the AATB-accredited laboratory collects the tissues from the hospital, processes them, and extracts the stem cells that will later be used to treat suffering patients in a clinic such as mine.

Umbilical cord tissue is regulated by the FDA guidelines that dictate the way human tissues can be harvested, stored, and utilized in treatment. According to Title 21 of the Code of Federal Regulations, these tissues must be "minimally manipulated" in order to be allowed in medical use. This means that they cannot be grown in a laboratory and then injected into the body. Instead, they need to be harvested directly from the umbilical cord, processed, and stored, ensuring their direct derivation from a human host.

The federal government's extensive regulations and oversight guarantees that patients scheduled for umbilical-cord stem cell therapy can rest easy, knowing the stem cells are safe and healthy. And unlike embryonic stem cells, umbilical-cord stem cells are not subject to ethical considerations. The parents get their healthy baby, and the "waste" product is used to treat patients suffering from persistent issues. It's a win-win situation!

WHAT MAKES UMBILICAL CORD STEM CELLS UNIQUE?

Unlike autologous stem cell therapy, in which the stem cells are derived from the patient's own adipose or bone marrow tissue, umbilical cord stem cells come from one of the most immature, healthy sources of stem cells available. As a result, these stem cells are remarkably potent and able to differentiate into a huge variety of key cells all over the body just as they would for a fetus in utero.

What's more, the umbilical cord contains Wharton's jelly, a gelatinous substance that insulates the blood vessels in the cord from damage. You can think of Wharton's jelly, an osteogenic substrate, as the body's natural lubricant, rich in stem cells that help regulate the natural motion of bones and joints. The cells that derive from Wharton's jelly enable the body to reconstruct bones and tissues. It's like building a firm foundation before pouring the concrete for a structure.

These distinctive properties of umbilical cord stem cells make the umbilical cord, in my opinion, the very best source of stem cells available. Their ability to differentiate into other types of cells and effectively regenerate the body's natural tissues make umbilical cord stem cell therapy the ideal treatment for a wide array of chronic pain disorders and diseases, including:

- arthritis,

- sports injuries,

- back, shoulder, hip, and knee pain,

- plantar fasciitis,

- fibromyalgia,

- multiple sclerosis,

- poststroke issues, and

- ALS.

It's high time that we stop throwing away umbilical cord and placental tissue and start utilizing the potent cells in this material to make chronic pain and disease things of the past for thousands of suffering patients all over the country. It's clear to me, to thousands of other clinicians like me, and to the hundreds of thousands of patients we've treated with umbilical cord stem cell therapy that this procedure is the future of medicine. But, you may ask, what does the procedure entail?

STEM CELL THERAPY VIA UMBILICAL CORD STEM CELLS

As mentioned earlier, umbilical cord stem cells are derived directly from the umbilical cord donated by the mother shortly after giving birth. If stored and banked properly, these cells are immediately ready for processing into stem cell treatments. The biological material is always thoroughly screened beforehand to check its viability and adherence to rigorous FDA guidelines that make sure the specimen has not been in any way compromised.

After these criteria have been met, the batch of processed rejuvenating stem cells can be delivered to the patient through an IV injection or by having them injected directly into the injury site. Since these stem cells are immune privileged, there is no risk of the patient's immune system rejecting the therapy. And as testament to the reliability of this procedure, over thirty thousand patients have undergone such treatments over the course of the past thirty-five years, without any known case of a major complication.

STEM CELL THERAPY VIA AMNION AND PLACENTAL TISSUE

Amniotic fluid is rich in growth factors and has stem cell qualities. Amniotic fluid injections are a cost-effective regenerative procedure that can be used for joint pain, in conjunction with other treatments or as a stand-alone treatment. The amniotic fluid product is an acellular cocktail of growth factors, peptides, and cytokines. It's harvested aseptically from planned cesareans and processed immediately via centrifugation, followed by a graduated freezing process.

No babies or fetuses are harmed in this process. The material is harvested from fluid that is normally thrown away. During the centrifugation process, all cellular material is removed and then it must go through a nine-step process of sterilization according to the FDA guidelines, which makes this one of the most sterile products on the market.

This product can be prepared frozen or dehydrated depending on the brand of amnion and there are different pros and cons to each, but both products are full of vital growth factors that aid in the body's natural healing process.

Amniotic fluid avoids the issue of patient variability and ensures a consistent level of bioactive growth factors at the time of injection. Once released, the 120-plus growth factors begin to recruit other endogenous regenerative cells and stem cells to the microenvironment where the growth factors are deployed, regardless of the patient's overall health.

Simply put, amniotic fluid helps anybody utilize regenerative medicine regardless of their health history. Amniotic fluid treatment simply involves the injection of the fluid into the joint or tendons as needed. This is done under the guidance of ultrasound or fluoroscopy to show the needle moving to the area of injury. We will discuss specific methods of deployment in more detail in the next chapter.

Chapter 7

THE DEPLOYMENT OF STEM CELLS AND REGENERATIVE CELLS

After stem cells have been sourced and undergone a thorough screening and vetting process to ensure they're safe, it's time for them to get to work in the patient's body. But how do they get in there? An autologous procedure uses stem cells that are processed that same day from the patient's own bone marrow or fat or are shipped from a cell banking facility, which we will mention later in the book. Allogenic cells from amnion, placenta, or umbilical-cord tissue will either be shipped overnight or taken from the clinic's onsite cell storage freezer.

Normally, an onsite freezer uses liquid nitrogen, according to a set of highly specific guidelines in order to keep tissues healthy and stable. Just prior to treatment, we thaw these tissues out and prepare them for use. Though we offer two at our clinic, there are four major strategies to implant the stem cells into the patient: (1) intravenous delivery, (2) intranasal delivery, (3) intra-articular delivery, and (4) delivery by nebulizer. But intravenous delivery is the simplest and most common method.

After administering light anesthesia if necessary (the treatment really doesn't hurt), we deploy (inject) the stem cells directly into the patient's bloodstream. As the stem cells move throughout the body, they secrete those cytokines we talked about before, which signal them to target damaged structures and begin differentiating, multiplying, and healing. For patients with systemic issues all over the body, such as rheumatoid arthritis or ALS, this procedure effectively gets the stem cells everywhere they need to go. The treatment takes about twenty to thirty minutes.

Intra-articular delivery is one of the most common procedures we offer in our practice because we primarily treat chronic pain. This procedure will be familiar to any patient who has ever received a cortisone shot or similar injection. For patients with deteriorating joints, we can inject stem cells directly into the problem area to get the joints working almost instantly. Even though stem cells have a homing property, they are injected as close to the area of injury as possible to ensure maximal efficacy. It's almost completely painless and achieves results within mere minutes. We will use imaging appropriate to the area where we are delivering the cells, which is the same way a traditional doctor administers a cortisone injection. For spinal areas, we use ultrasound imaging, which gives us a clear picture of small and medium-sized joints.

Ultrasound is a technology that doctors use to get a picture of the baby inside a pregnant mother. Ultrasound-guided injections are performed in much the same way as traditional injections are. To ensure the images are clear, an ultrasound gel is applied directly to the skin. The gel acts as a conductive medium that creates a tight bond between the skin and the ultrasound probe. This ensures the reflected sound waves are subjected to minimal interference. The probe, also known as a transducer, is placed near or adjacent to the targeted tendon or joint.

Once the doctor has identified the anatomic landmarks on the monitor, the injection will be delivered using a standard needle and syringe. That way, we are delivering the regenerative cells directly to the damaged area to maximize the healing benefits of this treatment.

Sometimes the type of procedure may warrant fluoroscopy imaging, which uses x-ray technology to create the image rather than the sound waves that ultrasound imaging deploys. The benefit of fluoroscopy is that it provides a clearer picture of the anatomy, but the disadvantage is that it uses low-dose radiation, which prevents it's use on pregnant women. Depending on the area where we are attempting to deliver the regenerative cells, we may utilize a contrast dye to pre-inject into the area to ensure we are within the capsule of the joint or the spinal region. While fluoroscopy itself is not painful, the particular procedure being performed may be painful, such as the injection into a joint.

Another quite common means of deployment is through the use of CT-guided injections. Computerized axial tomography (CT) is a common diagnostic tool that you may have had in the past, and this will provide the clearest and most precise image of surrounding anatomy. While you may be thinking that precise images are best, they are not as practical as the other methods we have used for years with an improvement in outcomes.

CT scans deliver much more radiation than fluoroscopy, and since CT machines are a much more expensive investment, our patients are treated by an interventional radiologist, which comes with a significant price tag. Generally, we use this type of deployment of stem cells when we need to pinpoint a specific area in the body. Overall, the CT deployment method is rarely used.

Intranasal delivery is an experimental strategy that is promising for patients with certain types of brain disorder, such as a recent stroke or multiple sclerosis. By going through the nose, we can deliver stem cells directly to the brain, encouraging the development of healthy brain tissues and thereby battling brain cancer and other hard-to-fight diseases.

Nebulizer delivery is another experimental procedure currently being tested in several studies. We hope stem cells that are nebulized and directly inhaled will be delivered to the lungs to address a wide variety of issues including lung cancer and chronic obstructive pulmonary disease (COPD). Trials on mice have been highly successful, though it may be a while before we start using this method on humans.

Regardless of how they are delivered, after the MSCs enter your body, they work in much the same way. The cytokines signal the cells to activate and make their way to your damaged tissues. Then, they begin to divide and differentiate. They spur widespread growth among dormant cells surrounding inflamed, injured structures by secreting proteins and recruiting growth factors in their mission.

They serve as the building blocks, multiplying over the next few weeks, which results in cascading benefits throughout the targeted area. The way stem cells work may be complicated, but the treatment and the results are as straightforward as they can be. And, typically, widespread beneficial effects are produced in just a few days after initial deployment.

Chapter 8

PREPARATIONS TO BE MADE BEFORE THE PROCEDURE

Before the stem cell procedure, we work to establish a healthy foundation for the stem cells to grow and thrive in. This means making sure that the patient is in a good state of mind prior to the cells' introduction. First, we coach the patient on stress management techniques. Persistent, overwhelming stress weakens the immune system and leads to all kinds of problem. In this chapter we will focus on reducing stress as well as making sure the body is at its best through diet and exercise.

TAKE SOME TIME FOR QUIET MEDITATION

First, we coach the patient on stress management techniques. We encourage many of our patients to meditate in the morning for just a few minutes, sitting down in silence and considering how they want their day to go. This helps them prepare for the day's challenges, sharpens focus and intention from the very beginning of the day, and, as studies show, generally boosts well-being over time.

GENERAL DIET RECOMMENDATIONS

Along with time for meditation and reflection, the food you eat before and after the procedure is also of tremendous importance. Your meals will provide the building blocks of nourishment for the stem cells in your body for months to come, so you might as well consider making some changes. There are many possible diets, but the consensus is that more vegetables are a good thing.

And don't worry about how many veggies to eat, because when it comes to vegetables, we can use all we can get. Just try to make leafy greens your number-one preference. They include spinach, chard, beet greens, kale, broccoli, and mustard greens, among others. This is the one area where almost all of us can improve our diet, and it is an especially important area of improvement for stem cell patients.

And when it comes to meat and other protein-based foods, we suggest patients eat small amounts of proteins frequently. It is best to have some protein at each meal, but not a large amount. In fact, it is best to stick to smaller amounts (less than two to four ounces of meat, fish, fowl, or eggs at a time). Both animal and vegetable sources of protein are beneficial. We understand that meat-and-potato eaters may find a plant-based diet too difficult to maintain, which is why we allow animal-based proteins as long as they're eaten in very small quantities.

Our advice is to choose a variety of meat products and find the healthiest options available (free-range, antibiotic-free and/or organic produce and products) whenever possible. Eggs, for most people, are an excellent source of protein. Eat the whole egg. The lecithin in the yolk is essential to lower blood fat and improve liver and brain function. The way in which you prepare a protein is critical. The closer you get to raw or rare-cooked food, the better, since the longer the food is cooked, the more nutrients it loses.

In fact, any time meats and vegetables are heated over 110° Fahrenheit, crucial enzymes are damaged and lost. Avoid frying. Grilling, boiling, steaming, soft-boiling and poaching are always the best methods. For vegetables, light steaming is your first choice. Sautéing is your second choice, and use only butter or olive oil to sauté.

Avoid iceberg lettuce for a salad and use lettuces with a rich green color. You also might want to eat sprouts and raw nuts. Just don't make salads your only choice for veggies. There are plenty of good greens you can eat, such as broccoli, spinach, and cucumbers. As for fruits, most people wrongly try to drink their fruits. This is a bad idea. Fruit juice is loaded with simple sugar fructose, which forms triglycerides and, ultimately, is stored as fat.

Without the fiber in the fruit, juice sends a rapid burst of fructose into the bloodstream. When you do eat fruit, only eat one type of fruit at a time, on an empty stomach. Avoid the sweetest fruits/tropical fruits, except papaya, which is very rich in digestive enzymes. Fruits from colder climates are preferable. In conclusion, eat only the highest-quality, fresh, and organic food whenever possible.

As you plan your diet, another thing to consider is your intake of carbohydrates. This is a very tricky area. Most people have one classification for carbohydrates when in reality there are really three different types: complex, simple, and processed. Unfortunately, for most patients suffering with imbalance problems, almost any carbohydrate is a no-no. It is a physiological fact that the more carbohydrates you eat, the more you will want. Craving carbohydrates is a symptom of an imbalance, so you can use this craving to monitor your progress.

Overall, eat vegetables as your carbohydrate choice and limit grains (even the whole grains can be trouble). When you do eat whole grains, only have them in moderation, and only at dinner. If you start the day with carbohydrates, you are more likely to crave them throughout the day, and then you'll eat more, and it's downhill from there.

There's another dark side to processed carbohydrates that isn't talked about much: their connection to weight gain, elevated cholesterol and triglycerides, heart disease, and cancer. To remain healthy, you really do need to limit your intake of high-carb foods, especially wheat and grains.

There has been a tremendous amount of debate regarding grains. Whole unprocessed grains can be rich sources of vitamins and minerals, but with soil depletion and the special strains of grain that modern agriculture has developed, it isn't clear what nutrients remain. The two grains predominantly used in this country are genetically engineered and have five times the gluten content and only one-third of the protein content of the original wheat from which they were derived.

This high-gluten content is to blame for many patients' allergic reactions. Unprocessed rye, rolled oats, and brown rice can be considered, *on occasion*, to give you more variety. But caution needs to be exercised when it comes to eating these foods on a regular basis. And 100 percent rye bread is the least of the evils. Stay away from white breads, muffins, cookies, candies, crackers, pastas, white rice, and most baked goods. Most importantly, your personal tolerance of gluten must be considered before adding it to your diet.

RECOMMENDATIONS FOR SWEETENERS AND OTHER ADDITIVES

Use only a small amount of raw honey or stevia as a sweetener. Absolutely no Nutra-Sweet, corn syrup, or table sugar should be used. An artificial sweetener such as Nutra-Sweet, in particular, contains aspartame, a chemical that can have damaging side effects. Although Nutra-Sweet still remains approved by the FDA, there is much scientific evidence that aspartame consumed over a long period of time can be a significant disruptor of the metabolism.

And ironically enough for all of you diet soda drinkers, that Nutra-Sweet in your diet soda could cause you to gain weight! The bad news is that as much as we all struggle to keep fat from accumulating in our midsection, we probably aren't consuming enough of the *right kinds of fats* in our diet in the first place. And what are the right kinds of fats?

Healthy fats can be obtained from dietary additives such as avocado oil, olive oil, walnut oil, flaxseed, raw nuts, and grape seed oils. These are all beneficial as long as they are cold-pressed. When cooking, use only raw butter, olive oil, or unrefined coconut oil. They are the safest oils to cook with. But avoid all hydrogenated and partially hydrogenated fats! They are poisons to your system. This means you should never eat margarine again. Also, avoid peanut butter (sorry, PB&J fans!). But by all means, eat all the avocados and raw nuts you desire.

RECOMMENDATIONS FOR DAIRY PRODUCTS

Forget pasteurized cow's milk products (milk, certain cheeses, sour cream, half and half, ice cream, cottage cheese, and yogurt). Believe me. If you knew all the potential problems caused by pasteurized milk, you would swear off it forever. Avoiding dairy will make it much easier for you to attain your optimal level of health and hormonal balance. Raw butter and kefir (liquid yogurt), however, are excellent sources of essential nutrients and vitamins. Raw goat's milk and sheep's milk cheeses and raw milk products in general are great alternatives.

Take a look at the table below for a list of foods we suggest you eat both before and after your stem cell procedure.

VEGETABLES	FRUITS	MEAT/ PROTEIN	ADDITIVES	BEVERAGES
artichokes	apples	beef	raw butter	bone broth
asparagus	bananas	caviar	sea salt	kefir
beans	most berries	chicken	black pepper	kombucha
beets	cantaloupe	fish	olive oil	milk
bell peppers	coconut	raw nuts	coconut oil	red wine
broccoli	lemons	organic pork	flaxseed oil	tea
cabbage	mango	lamb	apple cider dressing	vodka
cauliflower	oranges	duck		
celery	papaya			
chickpeas	pears			
cucumber	pineapple			
collard greens	pomegranate			
eggplant				
kale				
lentils				

VEGETABLES	FRUITS	MEAT/PROTEIN	ADDITIVES	BEVERAGES
lettuces				
okra				
zucchini				
Brussel sprouts				
sprouts				
mustard greens				
bok choy				
spinach				

AUTOIMMUNE CONDITIONS AND THE LEAKY GUT

One of the most common sources of inflammation in autoimmune patients and patients who eat the standard American diet is a condition called leaky gut syndrome. Though this disease is usually not recognized by the medical establishment, there's no shortage of evidence proving its existence.

When the tight junctions in your gut malfunction—usually because of inflammation or a disease such as celiac or Crohn's—the gut becomes more permeable than normal. This allows larger-than-normal particles to pass through your gut's walls and entering your bloodstream. And while this may sound innocuous enough, it's anything but, because your immune system targets them as intruders.

As a result, the immune system begins to exhaust its resources, essentially attacking itself. Whether patients have the telltale symptoms of leaky gut or are suffering from widespread autoimmunity problems. As we said before, stem cells are immunomodulating, which means they can boost a weak immune system or dampen an overactive one, but they can't accomplish this without the support of the rest of the body. Combining this type of therapy with dietary changes gives our patients the best possible outcomes.

Having that said, certain habits can depress or promote stem cell differentiation and growth after injection. And it is vitally important that patients focus on fostering patterns that promote tissue restoration and growth, which starts with removing the biggest sources of inflammation in their daily lifestyle. Smoking cigarettes and drinking are the most obvious culprits. There's no way to sugarcoat it: cigarettes and alcohol contain carcinogens that drastically and adversely disrupt the normal functioning of nearly all the body's systems, especially the immune system.

If you're drinking craft beer every night, or lighting up even once a day, you're just not going to reap the full benefits of stem cell therapy. We can tell you from our years in medicine that no matter the treatment, smokers and drinkers don't achieve outcomes as positive as those of healthier stem cell therapy patients. Routine drinking and smoking are not conducive to the success of stem cell therapy.

But do you know what is? Bone broth! Bone broth is an excellent health aid to healing and recuperation from illness. You've undoubtedly heard the old adage that chicken soup helps cure a cold. It turns out that scientific support for this adage exists. For starters, chicken contains cysteine, a natural amino acid that can thin the mucus in your lungs and make it less sticky so you can expel it more easily.

But there is a bit of a caveat to that, because processed, canned soups will not work as well as the homemade version made from slowly cooked bone broth. Medical scientists have discovered that overall health is in large part dependent on the health of the intestinal tract. Many of our modern diseases appear to be rooted in an unbalanced mix of microorganisms in our digestive system. Most of this affliction comes courtesy of an inappropriate and unbalanced diet that is way too high in sugars and too low in healthful fats and beneficial bacteria.

To borrow Dr. Natasha Campbell-McBride's term, bone broth is excellent for "healing and sealing" your gut. Dr. Campbell's GAPS nutritional protocol, described in her book *Gut and Psychology Syndrome* (GAPS), centers on the concept of gut health improved through diet. As her book indicates, broth, or stock, plays an important role in the health of the gut as it is easily digestible, helps heal the gut lining, and contains many valuable nutrients.

Bone broth helps to heal and seal the gut and promotes healthy digestion. The gelatin found in bone broth is a hydrophilic colloid. It attracts and holds liquids, including digestive juices, thereby supporting proper digestion. It also reduces joint pain and inflammation, courtesy of chondroitin sulfates, glucosamine, and other compounds extracted from the boiled-down cartilage. All of this serves to promote strong, healthy bones.

Bone broth contains high amounts of calcium, magnesium, and other nutrients that play an important role in healthy bone formation. Making your own bone broth is extremely cost effective, as you can make use of leftover bones that would otherwise be thrown away. And while the thought of making your own broth may seem intimidating at first, it's really quite easy. It can also save you money by reducing your need for dietary supplements.

Just to reiterate once again, bone broth provides you with a variety of important nutrients such as calcium, magnesium, chondroitin, glucosamine, and arginine that can save you a good deal of money. Instead of forking over your cash for these nutrients in the form of pricey health supplements, you can find everything you need in a good bowl of homemade bone broth.

Just make sure you use healthy ingredients such as grass-fed beef bones, free-range chicken (or much better, pasteurized chicken), and organic vegetables. You can also use a pressure cooker (such as an Instant Pot) instead of a slow cooker to dramatically reduce the cooking time. In recent years, Instant Pot has taken the world by storm with its ability to cook a wide variety of healthy foods in a short amount of time. Just about anything you can imagine can be cooked in Instant Pot, and it can be cooked well.

As you get ready to cook, you may want to consider the addition of vinegar. Not only are fats ideally combined with acids such as vinegar, but when it comes to making broth, the vinegar helps draw out all those valuable minerals from the bones and into the stockpot water that you'll drink. The goal is to extract as many minerals as possible from the bones into the broth water. Bragg's raw apple cider vinegar is a good choice, as it's unfiltered and unpasteurized.

In the end, however, these are just suggestions. There are lots of different ways to make bone broth and there isn't a wrong way to do it. You can find plenty of different variations online, but in order to give you a template with which to get started, we'll offer some basic directions. And as a side note, if you're starting out with a whole chicken, you'll have plenty of meat as well, which can be added back into the broth later, with extra herbs and spices, to make a chicken soup. We also use the chicken meat on salads.

Try these recipes:

CHICKEN BONE BROTH

Ingredients

1 whole free-range chicken, or 2–3 pounds bony chicken parts (necks, backs, breast bones, and wings)

gizzards from one chicken (optional)

2–4 chicken feet (optional)

4 quarts cold filtered water

2 tablespoons vinegar

1 large onion, coarsely chopped

2 carrots, peeled and coarsely chopped

3 celery stalks, coarsely chopped

1 bunch parsley

Main Directions

1. Fill a large stockpot (or large Crockpot) with pure, filtered water.
2. Add vinegar and all vegetables except parsley to the water.
3. Place the whole chicken or chicken carcass into the pot.
4. Bring to a boil and remove any debris that rises to the top.
5. Reduce the heat to the lowest setting and let simmer.

If you are cooking a whole chicken, the meat should start separating from the bone after about two hours. Simply remove the chicken from the pot and separate the meat from the bones. Place the carcass back into the pot and continue simmering the bones for another twelve to twenty-four hours. If you are cooking bones only, simply let them simmer for about twenty-four hours. Add the fresh parsley about ten minutes before finishing the stock, as this will add healthy mineral ions to your broth. Remove the remaining bones from the broth with a slotted spoon and pour the liquid through a strainer to remove any bone fragments.

BEEF BONE BROTH

Ingredients

4 pounds beef bones with marrow

4 carrots, chopped

4 celery stalks, chopped

2 medium onions, with peel, sliced in half lengthwise and quartered

4 garlic cloves, with peel and smashed

1 teaspoon kosher salt

1 teaspoon whole peppercorns

2 bay leaves

3 sprigs fresh thyme

5–6 sprigs parsley

¼ cup apple cider vinegar

18–20 cups cold water

Main Directions

1. Place all ingredients in a 10-quart slow cooker.
2. Bring to a boil over high heat; reduce and simmer gently, skimming the fat that rises to the surface occasionally.
3. Simmer for 24–48 hours.
4. Remove from heat and allow to cool slightly.
5. Discard solids and strain liquid through a colander into a bowl.
6. Let stock cool to room temperature, cover, and chill.
7. Use within a week or freeze up to 3 months.

Please take all of the recommendations presented in this chapter to heart so that you can have the best chance of success with your stem cell therapy. Sometimes just a little bit of change can make a big difference.

Chapter 9

COMPLICATIONS FROM LONG-TERM DRUG USE AND CONVENTIONAL TREATMENT

We have all heard the horror stories about the opioid crisis. Tales of withdrawal from an overdose of painkillers have flooded the airwaves. The victims come from all walks of life and share the same misfortune: a debilitating addiction to opioids.

Long-term opioid use can cause the following conditions:

1. *Memory problems.* Opioids have a direct impact upon the short-term memories of those who abuse them. One of the first symptoms of withdrawal is a severely disturbed memory and inability to process basic information. Opioids boost dopamine levels in the brain, bringing pain relief and an accompanying high. But the user quickly

overloads the brain's dopamine receptors, which disrupts the ability of the brain to store and create memory.

2. *Addiction.* Nowadays, addiction may seem like an obvious outcome of opioid use, but it isn't always so clear to the ones who end up addicted. As mentioned above, repeated opioid use stimulates the reward center of the brain, releasing dopamine into the system. These "happy chemicals" help to alleviate any pain and put the user in a permanently happy mood. The only trouble is that any chemical that artificially induces a feeling in the brain will only compromise the brain's ability to make that chemical on its own. It thus loses its capacity to create the right chemical balance needed and begins to depend on outside agents to keep itself functioning. In other words, the brain gets hooked on opioids. It's like that old commercial showing a whole raw egg in a pan, and an egg that gets scrambled as the narrator reads, "This is your brain—and this is your brain on drugs. Any questions?" There is no question that opioids can scramble our brains, leaving us with a pretty serious addiction.

3. *Constipation.* This is perhaps one of the lesser evils of opioid addiction, but it is a very common symptom nonetheless. Once introduced into the body, opioids immediately bind with opioid receptor proteins. These proteins are located in the brain along the spinal cord, and—yep, you guessed it—along the gastrointestinal tract. So, while the binding of opioid pain-relieving drugs with receptors along the spinal cord may be great for relieving back pain, the same binding that takes place in the gastrointestinal tract can

lead to constipation. Regular opioid use can also cause dehydration, exacerbating the problem even further and making it harder for the body to pass stool.

4. *Relationship issues.* The physical effects of opioid abuse are bad, but the effect it has on relationships are even worse. Those addicted to opioids have a hard time holding down jobs, interacting with spouses, taking care of kids—you name the relationship and opioid addicts will have issues with it. Opioid users may become so socially inept that they are unable to even make an appointment at a doctor's office. These relationship issues tend to spiral out into every facet of the opioid user's social life.

LONG-TERM INFLAMMATION TREATMENT

Inflammation has been under the microscope lately. Several research reports have begun to cite inflammation as a cause for everything from heart attacks and strokes, all the way to depression and anxiety. As such, many patients take medications and follow treatment plans to reduce the inflammation in their body. But these treatments can have adverse effects. So, let's go through some of the drugs prescribed, and conditions treated, for inflammation and the potential long-term ramifications of their use:

1. *Celebrex and heart attacks/strokes.* Celebrex is a particular brand of NSAID used for pain relief and chronic arthritis. As helpful as Celebrex may be, however, prolonged use can lead to chronic headaches, indigestion, anxiety, and insomnia. Even worse, Celebrex has been known to increase the risk of a heart attack and stroke. If patients

are experiencing such symptoms, they should discontinue their use of Celebrex and talk to their doctor.

2.   *NSAID use leads to internal bleeding and kidney disease.* Even general use of over-the-counter NSAIDs can cause a pretty major disruption of the body over time. At its worst, long-term use of NSAIDs can lead to bouts of internal bleeding and kidney disease. And at the very least, NSAIDs can interfere with stem cell treatment and should be avoided.

NON-OPIOID PAIN MEDICATION AND LIVER DISEASE

Many have tried to shift away from opioids to non-opioid medications, but long-term use of these can have their fair share of problems too. Most notably among them is liver disease. Here is a rundown of the most commonly used non-opioid pain medications and their effect on the liver.

1.   *Meloxicam.* This drug works by canceling enzymes that promote inflammation. Although highly effective in blocking inflammation, Meloxicam can lead to internal bleeding and stomach ulcers and adversely affect the liver and kidneys.

2.   *Acetaminophen.* This drug is another commonly prescribed medication for long-term inflammation treatment. But long-term use of acetaminophen can lead to liver disease and even liver failure.

3.   *Tramadol.* This drug is a pain reliever commonly used to treat moderate and severe pain in adults. It was originally designed as a nonaddictive pain killer, but over time, that

claim has proven to be incorrect. Drug abuse with this medication is not as common as with opioids, but the incidence of abuse is rapidly growing in the United States. Common side effects are headaches, dizziness, fatigue, constipation, diarrhea, nausea, stomach pain, anxiety, itching, and flushing.

COMPLICATIONS FROM GENERAL SURGERY

Although surgery is always a highly-scripted affair, the procedures are never perfect and there is always a risk of complication no matter what the procedure might entail. Any instance in which the skin is cut open automatically involves a level of risk. A blood clot, for example, would be a major complication, but residual, temporary pain is usually a minor complication of conventional treatment, whether it involves stem cells or not.

Chapter 10

ORTHOPEDIC PAIN

Anyone who has visited an orthopedics office knows that knee, shoulder, hip, back, neck, and muscular pain is big business. Patients who suffer from excruciating pain in these areas come from all walks of life including, among many others, construction workers who threw out their back and office clerks with a permanent kink in their neck. Chronic orthopedic pain is common. In this chapter, we will go over some of the main areas of orthopedic pain.

BACK AND NECK PAIN

The back and neck are among the most commonly reported sources of orthopedic pain. The joints of the neck and back are called facet joints. They serve to maintain the stability of the spine. They make sure that the spine is kept in proper alignment and not subjected to severe contortions. When functioning properly, these joints also serve to safeguard the vertebrae, preventing the incidence of a slipped disc, a painful condition in which one vertebra slips below another.

Complications of Back and Neck Surgery

As delicate as the back and neck are, every once in a while, complications are to be expected, especially if invasive surgery is involved. Here are a few of the most common.

1. *Complications of anesthesia.* Anesthesia is a great thing when it works as it is meant to, but there are times when pain-relieving anesthetics can go awry. Most surgeries involving the back and neck require some sort of general anesthesia. In some rare instances, patients could have an adverse reaction to the anesthetics they are given. It may be a direct reaction to the chemical compounds in the anesthetic, or it could be in relation to previous conditions that the patient had. Although extremely rare, complications caused by anesthesia have been known to occur.

2. *Failed-neck or back-surgery syndrome.* It is rather ironic that a procedure designed to eliminate back and neck pain could lead to further pain, but this is indeed a potential complication, and it is called failed-back-surgery syndrome. Some pain may be a temporary aberration that recedes in just a few days, but pain that persists longer than a few days needs to be addressed. If it is not addressed, the condition may deteriorate and lead to accumulation of scar tissue over spinal nerve roots, leading to even more chronic pain.

3. *Complications of fusion.* Although sometimes necessary, fusion can lead to quite a few complications. Number one

is its inability to alleviate chronic pain. Known as graft site pain, this pain sometimes has its origin in the bone graft itself. Fusion can also lead to the failure of the joints both above and below the area where the fusion took place.

4. *Risk of infection.* As with any surgery, the risk of infection is a rare possibility. But the risk of infection as a complication of back and neck surgery is so low that it is actually below 1 percent. The most common kind of infection occurs in the area of incision on the skin. An even rarer infection would involve the vertebrae or spinal cord. Antibiotics are often given before surgery in order to prevent complications from infection.

5. *Complications of epidural steroid injections.* Epidural steroid injections are given in order to alleviate pain and decrease inflammation. The epidural site of injection is in the region directly above the spinal cord and its accompanying nerve roots. One of the most serious complications occurs when a needle slips during administration and goes deeper than required, tearing a hole in nerve tissue, which leads to long-term neurological damage. Other potential long-term complications include an increase in headaches, localized pain, insomnia, and neurotoxicity.

6. *Hardware fracture.* In back and knee surgery, screws, plates, and rods are commonly used to hold vertebrae in place while everything heals after the procedure. This hardware can, on occasion, break down, leading to complications. When this happens, the hardware must be removed and replaced.

7. *Sexual problems.* This complication may come as a bit of a surprise, but both the back and the neck are connected to the spinal cord, and it is the nerves located inside the spine that facilitate crucial signals for sexual stimulation. Disruption of this communication can lead to sexual problems.

Common Conditions That We Treat with Stem Cells

Stem cells are on the cutting edge of treating back- and neck-based pain, and a wide variety of conditions can be treated.

1. *Degenerative discs.* Those who suffer from degenerative discs are faced with chronic neck, upper back, or lower back pain. MSCs have been shown to decrease the incidence of degenerative disc disease. These cells can work to rebuild broken-down connective tissues such as collagen, and help to rebuild the structure of the disc itself.

2. *Bulging discs.* Just as the term implies, a bulging disc forcibly bulges out of place. Conventional treatment requires surgical intervention that, basically, whittles down the bulge until it is no longer obtrusive. This may work as a quick fix, but in the long run, it simply makes the disc weaker, leading to even more problems. A culture of stem cells injected into the site of the bulge can directly heal and restore the damaged tissue that led to the bulge in the first place.

3. *Pinched nerves/sciatica.* Sciatica is a painful condition that afflicts many. It involves painful sensations felt up and down the sciatic nerve, whose nerve endings branch out from

the lower back and run down each leg. This condition is often caused when lumbar disc or bone pinches this nerve. Onsite injections of stem cells can help to restore these pinched nerves to their rightful state. We also perform the same procedure for pinched nerves in the cervical spine (neck).

4. *Arthritis.* Arthritic inflammation is a common cause of back and neck pain. Fortunately, it can be quite effectively treated with stem cells. Once injected, stem cells go right to the source of the inflammation and work to reduce it.

5. *Facet pain.* This is a condition in which the facet joints located on both sides of the spine have become disrupted. This could be due to acute injuries—for example, whiplash, or blunt force trauma—or the pain can come from slipped or bulging discs. An introduction of stem cells to the site of injury will help speed up healing and promote the regeneration of cartilage, tendon, and other tissues, which leads to the restoration of the facet joints to their rightful state. If you or someone you know received a radio-frequency ablation or a rhizotomy, there is a good chance they would benefit from a stem cell procedure in this area.

6. *Spinal steno*sis. Spinal stenosis occurs when there is a significant narrowing in the spaces of the spinal column. This constriction can lead to extra friction against the nerves that run up and down the spine. This narrowing is, generally, isolated to cases of cervical stenosis, related to the neck, and lumbar stenosis, related to the lower back. Symptoms include tingling, numbness, and pain. Stem

cell therapy has been shown to open up these constricted spaces of the spine, providing rapid relief for sufferers.

Stem Cell Treatments of the Joint

1. *Intradiscal injections.* All around the country, the deployment of stem cells to treat back and neck pain is subject to variation. Some doctors inject stem cells right into the disc (intradiscal injection) and some inject stem cells right to the edge of the disc (epidural injection). At our clinic, we have done both procedures but have recently discontinued injecting directly into the disc. We may change our mind in the future if we see more studies that support this protocol, but for the time being, we just haven't seen enough improvement to merit its continued use. Intradiscal injections are painful but do lead to improvement over time. However, we have not noticed an improved overall outcome compared to injecting right up to the disc, which is less painful.

2. *Epidural stem cell injection to the disc.* As mentioned above, epidural injection to the disc involves injecting stem cells just outside the disc. We have found that deploying (injecting) the stem cells much like an epidural, right to the outer disc wall, works best. This method of deployment allows the stem cells to be better drawn to the damage and tears in the disc, which is the reason why it bulged in the first place. The wall of the discs between the vertebrae comprises a series of rings around a "jelly donut" in the middle of the disc, and when the wall is weakened, the jelly will push out toward the weakened area. If the patient

is lucky, the bulge pokes into nothing. If the patient is unlucky, it pushes on a spinal nerve or the spinal cord. If it pushes on a spinal nerve, it will cause shooting pain down the arms or legs, but if it pushes on the spinal cord, it will cause spinal stenosis symptoms. Having that said, we have found that we get the best results when we supply the stem cells right to the walls of the disc, and then follow up the treatment with spinal decompression therapy. This is much like traction therapy, which creates a negative pressure so the disc pulls away from the nerve. It also gives the stem cells a chance to start rebuilding the outer wall of the disc, which will eventually allow the bulge to stay away from the nerves and cause no further problems for the patient.

3. *Recommended physical therapy.* We have many patients who tried physical therapy for their spinal conditions and failed to see results. When patients suffer from one of these underlying conditions, just strengthening a few muscles most likely won't be enough to eliminate their pain. As cartilage starts to regrow between the spinal joints, patients will need to strengthen the surrounding muscles again. Our program looks at the joints above and below the area of complaint. We try to make sure that these joints and muscles are moving properly, because this motion is vital for the joints to start healing. Next, we strengthen weak muscles all around the vertebrae, which means on the front side and on the back side. It's a little more complicated than I'm letting on, but any rehabilitation specialist should be able to accomplish this, and the beauty of this therapy is that in most cases it is covered by insurance. Patients will usually get the best results from a sports medicine

chiropractor or manual physical therapist. These types of providers address muscular fascia problems through a type of massage. They address fixated joints and reinforce the change through rehabilitative exercises. Usually, they can be found in the sports community. We find they are the best equipped therapists to handle this kind of pain problem, and we employ them for the physical therapy we recommend to our patients after the stem cell procedure.

4. *Light therapy, laser therapy,* or *PEMF therapy.* We have a separate chapter devoted to this topic, but it is important to stress here its importance for stem cell treatments of the back and neck joints. Many of our spinal patients require one of these types of therapy in order to accelerate the proliferation of the stem cells in the spine. We always want maximum growth from our stem cells, but we especially want to make it a top priority in spinal procedures because we know that if our treatment should fail, the only alternative would be surgery. We make every attempt to have all of our patients avoid surgery because spinal surgeries have by far the poorest rate of successful outcome. Interestingly, we have treated the spinal problems of many physicians with this combination of stem cell therapy and therapy that accelerates stem cell proliferation. The reason for our popularity with physicians may be that they know better than anyone else that surgery has a poor success rate as a treatment for spinal conditions. Most important, however, is that coupling stem cell treatment with one of the above-mentioned cell-proliferation therapies is imperative to ensure a speedy and successful recovery.

BONNIE T.'S STORY

Bonnie was one of our patients who suffered from the outcome of a motor vehicle accident. Bonnie was involved in a traumatic accident twenty-two years before she came to our office and she'd had emergency surgery for her spine. When one area of her spine was fused together, the areas above and below her fusion began to pick up excess movement. This led to degenerative disc disease above and below her surgery site and she suffered sacro-iliac pain. The sacro-iliac joint is the pelvic joint, which can cause buttock pain if it is injured. Bonnie was referred to our office by her pain management physician, who had run out of options for her. She had already consulted several surgeons who did not want to operate on her, because they couldn't guarantee that she would get better. She had exhausted all of her other options, though. Over the years, she had received hundreds of acupuncture, chiropractic, physical therapy, massage, and other treatments. She had tried cannabinoids, pain creams, burning of the nerves, and implantable neurostimulation devices, and she was taking strong opioid pain killers. Her quality of life was decreasing because she couldn't sleep, she couldn't walk for exercise, and she continued to suffer from what she was told were just worn-out arthritic joints (degenerative discs and sacro-iliac joints).

Bonnie wasn't ready to throw in the towel at such a young age. She was active, involved in many activities in the community, and didn't let pain get in her way. Although every morning was a struggle for her, she didn't want pain to be the major motivator of all of her decisions in life.

When her pain management physician told her he had run out of options and suggested she consider stem cell treatment, he referred her to our office. With a couple of injections of stem cells into the areas around the fusion and her sacro-iliac joint, she was able to walk again within one week. She was so impressed with this type of therapy that she returned two years later to receive stem cells in her knees and had some extra adipose cells shipped off to a laboratory to be used for future treatments.

Bonnie wasn't scared of surgery, but she knew that surgical complications could be fatal or at the very least permanent, which is why she opted for stem cells for the future. She had no downtime, and with some therapy treatment and physical therapy strengthening after her treatment, she had her life back. She is a big stem cell advocate and has spoken to many people in her community about this treatment and how it saved her life.

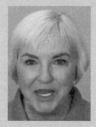

Bonnie T., retired, CA—degenerative discs disease, sacro-iliac and post surgical pain

GUS S.'S STORY

Gus was a hard-working man and business owner who wasn't going to let back pain get in his way. He managed it with injections and new procedures such as radial frequency ablations, which eliminated his pain for years. But time was beginning to catch up with him. He suffered from multiple disc bulges pushing on his spinal cord, which gave him spinal stenosis and was combined with arthritis in his facets.

When the spinal cord is subjected to pressure, it can cause radiating pain down the legs and back pain as well, and it usually makes the legs feel weak. At first, the steroid injections managed to control Gus's pain, but over a span of two years, his pain progressed. He had to give up golf, which he loved, but he just accepted that deprivation as part of aging. When, finally, he came to our office, he was assisted into the waiting room.

He was unable to drive or stand on his own for very long, and he was desperate for a solution. His steroid shots were not working anymore, and his spine surgeon told him that surgery would result in a 50 percent chance of his ending up in a wheel chair for the remainder of his life and a 50 percent chance of his getting better.

His cardiologist was very much against surgery because Gus would have to stop taking the blood thinner the cardiologist had prescribed to prevent another heart attack or a stroke. Gus would have to stop taking the blood thinner for some time after such major surgery in order to allow his body to heal.

Fortunately for Gus, his neighbor was researching stem cell therapy and already had a copy of the previous edition of our stem cell book, which he gave to Gus. After reading the book, Gus discussed the therapy with his wife and decided he should try it before rolling the dice on surgery. He knew he didn't have a choice anymore, because he couldn't even go the bathroom without assistance. He sat in a recliner all day because he couldn't move, and to add insult to injury, all of his friends and family golfed, but he couldn't even stand on his own.

Gus's first session in our California office took a long time because, due to his back spasms, just getting him into various positions for examination took many minutes. We decided that Gus would need the works. He was evaluated for his physical therapy protocol, and ten areas in his lower spine, each bulging disc, and each arthritic facet were treated. Then he started a series of spinal decompression therapy sessions in which negative pressure was put on his damaged discs, which received laser treatments. He had joint mobilization therapy to restore normal alignment, and he started physical therapy at the end of the first month.

He was put on a weight loss program because overweight people have a build-up of fat in the spinal canal. Losing weight was also good for his heart. The program took close to four months to complete, but at the end of it, not only was Gus out of pain but he was also golfing again for the first time in two and a half years.

Gus was a very compliant patient and worked very hard, and he was grateful he had been given a second shot at life again. His wife was also extremely happy because they could now sleep together, he could go to the bathroom on his own and drive on his own, and she got her old husband back. She wasn't ready to become a caretaker. Many times, we forget that our chronic pain puts a burden on our family members.

Some patients are concerned with the cost of therapy, but if they calculate the cost of a caretaker and the burden put on their spouse and the children, the therapy is much more economical. Gus's family just wanted him to be pain-free and happy again.

Complete 180-degree-turnaround stories such as Gus's are not uncommon with this type of therapy, but complicated cases like his require a multipronged approach, which is why we offer a multidisciplinary approach.

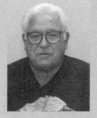

Gus S., business owner, OR—spinal stenosis and arthritis

SHARON S.'S STORY

We give many of our spinal treatments to patients suffering as a result of an old car accident, just as Sharon did. She is a retired pharmacist whose car was rear-ended in 1973 by a truck driver. In the past, vehicles didn't have air bags, crumple zones, and adequate seat belts, which led to many whiplash-related injuries.

The vertebrae are connected by ligaments that include intervertebral discs and ligaments running along the front, back, and even the facet joints. When you are hit at a high speed, your bones are stretched passed their normal limits, which creates permanent laxity in the ligaments that hold the vertebrae together. Many times, the capsules that hold the facets together and also hold synovial fluid in the joints have microtears that create a constant, dull, ache in the muscles of the upper shoulders (trapezius and levator scapula). Patients feel better when they have their neck stretched or after physical therapy exercises, but the ache builds up again by the end of the day.

Sharon was able to manage this pain with injections, chiropractic, physical therapy, and massage until 2004, when she received cervical decompression and fusion surgery. The excess mobility and damage to her cartilage reached a point where the pain was severe, and she developed shooting pain down her arms. She had surgery to address some of the arthritis and stabilize the area, using rods and pins between two vertebrae.

She received relief from the surgery. However, when one area of the spine is stabilized, the areas above and below the fusion in the spine become destabilized. In her late seventies, Sharon wasn't as optimistic about receiving another fusion surgery in 2018, which is why she sought out stem cell therapy. Being a pharmacist, she had researched her alternatives to this treatment and didn't wish to proceed with the traditional treatment of burning the nerves, controlling the pain, and eventually, fusing another area. Sharon had worked hard her entire life so she could have choices later in life, and she determined that a major surgery at her age wasn't a good idea. Plus, she knew the recovery would likely take longer than a year.

Her procedure was very simple: We suggested she receive a treatment that combined a mixture of stem cells from her fat with growth factors from amniotic fluid. Most of her pain came from her facet joints above and below her fusion, and one of her discs between the vertebrae was also generating some pain. We treated the facets above and below her joint and the disc with the injections, which were administered under fluoroscopy, providing a crystal-clear image of her spine. The injections were no more painful than an epidural, which she had had previously and which was no longer alleviating her pain.

It took her close to five months to get 100 percent of pain relief from this treatment. She also received laser treatments to stimulate the growth of the stem cells after the treatment, which allowed her to start feeling some relief by her second month. She also started physical therapy exercise in her second month. Overall, we have found this protocol to be the most complete.

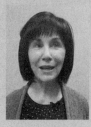

Sharon, S., retired pharmacist, CA—arthritis and cartilage damage

KNEE PAIN

Ada's Story

My name is Ada, and every winter, my family and I head to the mountains for a week to decompress from the madness of the holiday season. I love this time of year, and as an avid skier, I look forward to few things more than making fresh tracks. This was my thirty-first consecutive winter of skiing, and I was armed with a backpack of water and protein bars so I didn't have to waste a minute of the day. My son and I warmed up on a few runs and then took the lift to our favorite black diamond run on fresh powder.

We began our descent, and I easily kept pace with my athletic teenage son, but just as we rounded a soft bend in the run, a skier blasted out of the trees to my right and slammed into me. That is the last thing I remember before waking up at the bottom of the hill on a stretcher. I had been knocked unconscious, and the ski patrol had carefully transported me to the first-aid station to await an ambulance.

My first thought was to wonder if the other skier was okay, but my second thought quickly focused on my knee. All I could feel was excruciating pain and burning. My son was next to me, and I soon saw my daughter and husband ski up to the stretcher. Their faces expressed fear. I reassured them that I was okay, and they reassured me that the other skier was just a little banged up.

Over the next few weeks, the reality of what happened sunk in more deeply with every doctor's appointment. I had a combo injury that orthopedists refer to as the unhappy triad. The force of the collision with the other skier had sprained my knee, causing injury to my right anterior cruciate ligament (ACL), medial collateral ligament (MCL), and meniscus.

Doctors were unwavering: I needed surgery, medications for pain, and physical therapy. In the meantime, I was relegated to minimal movement and a very sedentary life. I had numerous friends who had undergone new surgeries with poor results, and I was hesitant to do something that could make my knee worse. So, before I decided to go under the knife, I asked around and did some research. I am so glad that I did because the results I had from non-invasive surgeries, harnessing my own body's innate healing, have given me back a healthy knee and the ability to hit my thirty-second season on the slopes.

Healing without Surgery

Ada came to our office committed to avoiding surgery, but her injuries were severe. She was in great health and had been an athlete her whole life, so she was no stranger to putting in the work that was needed to meet her goals. Ada wanted to understand the anatomy of her knee and how the therapies offered might help her mend. The patients who better understand how their bodies work and heal have the greatest commitment, and therefore success, after treatment. Let's take a quick dive into the anatomy of the knee and how Ada's injuries set her up for a tricky recovery.

Inside the Human Knee

The femur, tibia, patella, and fibula are the bones that come together to make up the knee. The knee operates primarily as a hinge joint but retains some ability to rotate as well. It is filled with synovium, a special lubricating fluid that ensures that bone and cartilage do not grate against each other during movement. Articular cartilage caps off the ends of the femur and tibia. The joint can become arthritic if this cartilage is injured.

The knee has the following components:

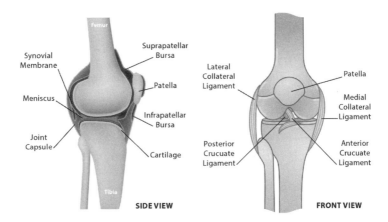

Synovial Membrane — *Femur* — *Suprapatellar Bursa* — *Patella* — *Meniscus* — *Infrapatellar Bursa* — *Joint Capsule* — *Cartilage* — *Tibia*

SIDE VIEW

Lateral Collateral Ligament — *Patella* — *Medial Collateral Ligament* — *Posterior Crucuate Ligament* — *Anterior Crucuate Ligament*

FRONT VIEW

- *Bones.* Connecting the femur bone of the thigh and the tibia bone of the shin is the largest and most complicated joint in the human body, the knee.

- *Ligaments.* The knee joint, containing the patella (knee cap) and adjacent bones, is held together by the medial collateral ligament (MCL), the lateral collateral ligament (LCL), the anterior cruciate ligament (ACL) and the posterior cruciate ligament (PCL).

- *Cartilage.* Situated between the bones is a crescent-shaped disc of cushioning cartilage that stabilizes the joint called the meniscus. The meniscus helps to protect the joint from wear and tear but is vulnerable to tearing, especially in older adults.

- Articular cartilage acts as a shock absorber and is found on the femur, the top of the tibia, and the back of the patella. It also helps bones move over each other without friction.

- *Joint capsule.* Surrounding the joint is a membrane sac that contains a liquid called synovial fluid, which lubricates and nourishes the joint.

- *Bursa.* There are over a dozen, tiny, fluid-filled sacs in the knee joint. They prevent friction and inflammation. However, if they do become inflamed, a painful condition called bursitis can occur.

Living with Knee Pain

Especially as we age, knee injuries are not uncommon, because the knee joint is under pressure and in use most of the time. Whether we are sitting, standing, running, walking, squatting, or moving in any direction, the knee is, typically, involved and taking the brunt of the load. While the knee joint is large, it's also vulnerable. One wrong twist or bend can damage the many important tissues in the knee, affecting all the other components as well.

It's not just trauma that can damage a knee. Repetitive movements are also a risk factor for knee injury. Whether it's a faulty golf swing, a slightly imbalanced running gait, or even athletic overuse, seen regularly in the CrossFit community, the knee can wear down over time and lead to painful and degenerative symptoms. The most common knee injury impacts the ACL, estimated to affect one in every 3,500 people in the USA—that is, between 100,000 and 200,000 people each year.

Knee pain can be extremely challenging to live with. For the same reasons that knee injuries are so common, the resulting pain is difficult to manage. This is because knees are in constant use. Even when we are sitting down, the knee must bend, which alleviates pressure on one area while increasing pressure on another. Most often, my patients report the pain is so restrictive that they've been forced to reduce their activity levels and avoid so many things they used to enjoy including traveling, hiking, dancing, or simply walking. Losing the ability to engage in the activities that we love is not only physically damaging but mentally and emotionally damaging as well.

Even giving up favorite activities does not mean pain relief for most people. So many resort to using pain medications to manage the symptoms. Whether you're using NSAIDs such as ibuprofen or prescription drugs, this is not a good long-term solution. Any pain medication has dangerous and, sometimes, lasting side effects. Worse, masking the pain can lead to unknowingly overuse of the vulnerable knee, exacerbating injuries and symptoms.

Conventional Counsel

In the conventional health care system, doctors counsel their patients that the alternative to pain management is surgery. Surgery is not something to be taken lightly or rushed into. In fact, knee surgery can have long-term side effects and is definitely not guaranteed to be successful. One of the most common complications, often overlooked, especially when a patient is young, is postoperative arthritis. Surgery around joints increases the risk of arthritis later, which increases the chances of another surgery. In fact, the risk of developing osteoarthritis is three times more likely after the common ACL reconstructive surgery.

Knee surgery is traumatic to surrounding tissues, which can cause depletion of cartilage and the shrinking of space between the knee components, leading to more friction and less stability. So, the immediate injury might be improved by surgery, but surgical side effects bring about their own nasty symptoms. Especially as we age, decreased stability of the knee means a higher risk of secondary injuries and falling.

A Fear of Falling

Falling is not to be taken lightly. For the elderly, falling is the leading cause of fatal injury. Shockingly, every twenty minutes in the USA, an older adult dies from injuries related to falling. Treating fall-related injuries in 2013 cost the health care system over $34 billion, and that number is expected to increase to over $67 billion in 2020. Something to keep in mind is that falls are seven times more likely for unhealthy adults than for those who prioritize their health.

So, when unhealthy older adults take a fall, it's often the beginning of the end. Their bodies struggle to recover, and they regularly experience a steeper decline in health. While the fall might have triggered the decline, it is not uncommon for other fatal illnesses to result. After a fall, the recovery period and the use of prescription pain medications can weaken the immune system and cause unforeseen psychological damage. Some studies explain that fall anxiety can prevent elderly people from participating in activities, so instead of getting out and staying active, they resign themselves to sedentary and isolating behavior.

Even if we ignore the risk of arthritis, additional surgeries, falling, or the reality that recovery from some surgeries takes at least three months and often longer, surgery is not guaranteed to work. Few patients think of asking their surgeon how successful the procedure is likely to be, because they assume their doctor wouldn't put them under the knife if it weren't going to work. All patients should ask their doctors for the rate of success and how they're measuring the success of any procedure. The reality is that surgery may not yield better outcomes than doing nothing at all.

The *New England Journal of Medicine* published a study in 2013 by Finnish researchers who looked at the effects of arthroscopic partial meniscectomies to repair meniscus tears, the most frequent orthopedic surgery performed in the USA. There were 146 participants between the ages of thirty-five and sixty-five, and they were divided into two groups. One group received genuine surgery and the other group received sham surgery.

The study concluded that "resection of a torn meniscus has no added benefit over sham surgery to relieve knee catching or occasional locking. These findings question whether mechanical symptoms are caused by a degenerative meniscus tear and prompt caution in using patients' self-report of these symptoms as an indication for APM."

Every participant in the study had surgery, but half of them did not get genuine surgery. Regardless of whether they had the actual arthroscopic partial medial meniscectomy or a placebo surgery, the results were the same. The real surgery provided *no significant benefit*! Researchers warn that we must rethink whether meniscus damage is the true cause of the symptoms that doctors address with surgery.

Meniscus surgeries are not the only concern. Up to 15 percent of ACL surgeries leave patients with unsatisfactory results and require a secondary surgery. Revision surgeries are problematic because their rate of success is even lower. The goal of orthopedic surgery is usually the improvement of the patient's quality of life, whether that involves pain reduction or increased mobility.

However, a study published in the *British Journal of Medicine* in 2017 concluded that knee replacement surgeries did not yield significant improvements in quality of life. In fact, in the group of almost five thousand participants, only those with the most severe knee conditions felt that their surgery was a success. The study concluded that knee replacement should be reserved for only the most severely affected patients if the health care system would like to see better success rates from surgery.

Surgery as a Last Resort

Surgery is the standard of care for these injuries, but we should not jump to these expensive and risky procedures without exhausting much less expensive, less risky, and less costly options. At the very least, providers should educate their patients about every evidence-based option available so they can make an informed decision.

It's easy to be skeptical about the road less traveled, and maybe, if we had not seen so many people improve and recover from knee injuries and a variety of other severe conditions without surgery, we would not believe there was another way. However, not only have countless patients left our office in full recovery after noninvasive treatments, but some physicians have also experienced the benefits as well.

Healing a Knee with Stem Cells

While stem cells can be injected throughout the body, and they are brilliant at finding the areas that need healing, we give them some help by injecting them directly into the injury zone in the knee joint. This is beneficial because the reduced blood flow in joints makes it more difficult for stem cells to reach the target tissues.

Injecting directly into the site is delicate work because we want the stem cells to be placed correctly, but we don't want to cause any additional agitation or injury. That is why it still surprises me that some providers inject stem cells without using live imaging, relying instead on old still images of their patient's knee.

This is why we find it imperative to use live imaging, because with the use of ultrasound or fluoroscopy. This allows us to see exactly what is happening in the knee as we carefully inject the cells. We use this type of imaging for any injection into the knee, including stem cells, PRP, or Hyalogen (hyaluronic acid) so the procedure has optimal precision.

Because stem cells trigger repair cells to kick into action, results can happen quite quickly, but they may take anywhere from eight weeks to six months to be fully effective. We have seen a range of timelines, depending on patients' health at the time of the procedure and how they care for their body afterward. Because results vary, depending on the extent of the injury and the patient's overall health and age, we use additional therapies and post-care guidelines to give our patients the best results. Occasionally, a patient's results exceed our expectations and leave us in awe. My mom was one of those patients.

In her late sixties, she still actively runs a business, exercises regularly, and enjoys taking dance classes. So, one day, when she heard a "pop" in her knee and became instantly debilitated, she was scared. She went to her regular physician and was given pain medication, but after a week or so, her condition had not improved. Her doctor recommended an orthopedic specialist who soon concluded that she'd torn her meniscus. He told her that because she already had some age-related arthritis, she would benefit from arthroscopic surgery and, later, a knee replacement.

Throughout this time, I was kept in the dark. My mom didn't want to bother me, so I was shocked when she finally shared that she was considering knee surgery. Obviously, I objected and quickly began a series of PRP injections—the therapy that world-class athletes such as Kobe Bryant, Tiger Woods, and Alex Rodriguez have benefited from—while supporting her weakened knee with a brace. We also used knee decompression therapy, which helps to open the joint, alongside stem cell injection to regrow the knee tissue and space.

In less than a month, my mom was moving, dancing, and working as if nothing had happened. She is a rock star among her friends, many of whom have had knee surgeries without half of the success of my mother's. But she is not a miracle patient. She represents a large population of people who successfully respond to non-invasive procedures that help them avoid surgery.

Truth be told, my mom was blown away and grateful for her results. So later, when the osteoarthritis that had been developing in her hand for over twenty years eventually crippled her mobility, we tried again. She received a stem cell injection into the hand that was stuck in a permanent claw shape, and within thirty minutes, she had nearly a full range of motion.

You might be tempted to think that my mom is somehow unique, or maybe just has good healing genes. Genetics are a factor, but so is our general state of health. The healthier the body is at the time of any procedure, the greater the likelihood of getting the best results. Genetics are not carved in stone. In fact, our genes are continuously turned on and off by environmental factors such as nutrition, exercise, toxic exposure, hydration, and stress. So, if we harness the power of lifestyle and environment to improve our health and healing, the outcome is always better.

One of the reasons that we are so successful with stem cell treatment in our clinic is because we pay close attention to the health of the patient and their injured joint before and after stem cell injection. Whether we're treating arthritis, meniscus, or tendons and ligaments such as the ACL, boosting the body's ability to repair is critical for success. Not only do we use therapies that improve the effectiveness of stem cells but we also educate our patients with detailed post-care instructions to ensure their health improves rather than diminishes throughout the healing process.

HIP PAIN

The hip, as is the shoulder, is a ball-and-socket joint. The socket is the acetabulum, and the femoral head makes up the ball. The hip brings the femur and pelvis together to create this major weight-bearing joint. The ball joint is attached to the socket by ligaments. This joint is covered by synovial fluid, as is the knee. The muscles connected to the hips are the hamstrings, quadriceps, iliopsoas muscle, gluteal, and abductor muscles.

Complications of Hip Surgery

Hip replacement surgery comes with a whole host of potential complications and risks. Some of them are more troubling than others.

Here is a list of the most common complications.

1. *Blood clots.* It is said that about one out of every hundred patients who have hip surgery end up suffering a venous thromboembolism, otherwise known as a blood clot. These clots seem to occur whether patients are sent home after surgery or have an extended stay in the hospital.

2. *Nerve damage.* There is now plenty of research out there to indicate that, immediately following hip surgery, subsequent inflammation can lead to nerve damage. This

can then progress into chronic neurological conditions such as neuropathy.

3.   *Infection.* It is true the threat of infection can be present in just about any procedure, but there is a repeated incidence of infection occurring after hip replacement surgery. Usually, the infection is caught fairly early and the physician is able to inject antibiotics and clear it out. But if the infection persists, the implant from the hip replacement procedure may need to be removed. In the absolute worst cases of post-procedure infection, the affected hip, as well as the whole leg may be subject to amputation.

4.   *Dislocation.* Although rare, on some occasions the implanted replacement becomes dislocated after hip surgery.

5.   *Incongruent leg length.* This potential complication is just about as alarming as it sounds—but it does happen. There are some incidences of patients ending up with one leg shorter than the other after hip replacement surgery.

6.   *Pain.* Pain, of course, is the most common postsurgical complication and can vary in severity. For most, the pain only lasts a day or so and quickly subsides. For others however, the pain might persist for weeks or even months. One large study showed that as much as 27 percent of total-hip replacement patients continued to experience varying degrees of postsurgical pain for three to four years after surgery. The persistent pain was most commonly described as aching, tender, and tiring. Now a new study questions that efficacy even further, showing that only about half of the patients who get a knee or hip replaced have significant improvement in pain and mobility after the

surgery. The authors of the study looked at 2,400 patients with both common and inflammatory arthritis. Nearly 480 of these patients had a knee or hip replacement, and of the 202 patients included in the study, only half reported, one to two years after surgery, a meaningful improvement in their hip and knee pain and disability. What's more, researchers found that the patients who were more likely to report benefit were those who had suffered the worst knee or hip pain before surgery but had fewer general health problems and no arthritis besides the arthritis that was in the joint before it was replaced. Nearly 83 percent of study participants had at least two troublesome knees and/ or hips. In general, an estimated 25 percent of patients who undergo a single joint replacement will have another joint replacement within two years. This fits with what we see in the clinic because most of our patients have pain in multiple areas. So, to conclude, I would have to say that these very invasive surgeries often fail to satisfy the clinical expectations of patients. If you have pain in multiple areas, the results of a knee or hip replacement surgery may be disappointing.

7. *Decreased activity.* The belief that a hip replacement will increase your activity level is another incorrect impression that needs to be debunked. That 2013 study on activity levels after a total hip replacement is a meta-analysis, which means that it compiled and analyzed many earlier studies—in this case seventeen. Included are studies that provide measurements of physical activity prior to hip replacement, and up to one year following it. The meta-analysis concludes that "there is no statistically significant

difference in physical activity levels before and up to one year after unilateral primary total hip replacement." And supporting this conclusion are other studies on activity levels following hip replacement. One on jogging, for example, shows that if you aren't jogging prior to your hip replacement, it's unlikely you will jog following your hip replacement. Those who don't jog prior to the surgery but who hope to begin jogging after it found it impossible, due a number of issues: pain, anxiety, decreased range of motion, muscle weakness, and low back or knee pain. In addition, only 70 percent of those who jogged prior to their hip replacement did so after it. As a result of all this, some patients actually lost ground instead of gaining it. The upshot? If you aren't biking, jogging, or climbing mountains before you have a hip replacement, it's highly unlikely you'll suddenly be more active after hip replacement. But even if you are doing these things prior to surgery, there's a good chance you'll never get back to the activity level you are enjoying now! And to make matters worse, throw into the mix the continued struggles with pain following hip replacement, and the serious risks involved. At any rate, understanding the wrong impressions you may have about hip replacement should help you come to the right decisions when considering this surgery.

Common Conditions That We Treat with Stem Cells

In this section, we will discuss some of the conditions of the hip that are most commonly treated with stem cells.

1. *Chronic bursitis.* Chronic bursitis is a condition in which a bursa, a fluid-filled sac that cushions joints such as the hip, bursts open. This rupture is usually caused by repetitive motion. The onset of the condition in the hip can be caused simply by walking. Blunt force is another cause. For example, if you were to fall down in a parking lot, slamming your hip hard, the bursa could be disrupted. This condition can be treated with a simple onsite injection of the patient's own specially prepared stem cells.

2. *Osteoarthritis.* This is a very common condition and one of the most successful conditions to be treated with stem cells. Osteoarthritis is a degenerative joint disease, and since stem cell therapy is a restorative method of treatment, it can get right to the root of the problem. Stem cells lock on to the damaged and degenerative tissue and immediately begin rebuilding and repairing them back to a normal state.

3. *Labral tears.* Hip labral tears occur when the labrum, a band of cartilage surrounding the hip joint, is injured. Labral injuries can be the result of trauma, such as a fall or a car accident, but are most commonly caused by repetitive trauma to the hip joint. Individuals who participate in sports that require extremes of motion, such as long-distance running or figure skating, or require repetitive twisting and "cutting," such hockey or soccer, are most often diagnosed with labral tears. The typical patient we treat has failed to benefit from physical therapy and cortisone injections and does not want hip surgery. Depending on the patient's age, a hip surgeon may recommend a total hip

replacement, which is why many labral tear sufferers seek stem cell therapy.

Stem Cell Treatment of the Joint

1. *Injection into the joint under imaging.* In this procedure stem cells are procured from the patient, processed, and delivered right into the joint via advanced guided imagery. This method enables the attending physician to pinpoint the exact site of injection as well as more effectively control the direction in which the stem cells are injected into the patient.

2. *Recommended physical therapy.* Physical exercise after treatment is highly recommended. Walking, riding a stationary exercise bike, using an elliptical machine, or swimming are all good forms of physical therapy. The patient should avoid activities that might be too strenuous, such as running or intensive sports.

3. *Key areas to strengthen.* Key areas to strengthen after the procedure are the gluteal muscles (buttocks) and the lower abdominals, which form a natural support structure for the hips, stabilizing them and helping them to function correctly. The stronger these muscles are, the better the hips will function.

SPECIFIC PROCEDURES FOR SPECIFIC CONDITIONS

Before   **After (4 Months)**

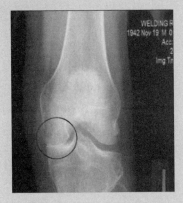
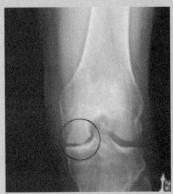

Some patients may see a visible change on their x-ray images, such as in the images shown above, but not everyone will have a visible change after one treatment. However, most will experience a decrease in their pain level or complete elimination of their pain after one treatment. In fact, most orthopedic conditions will have between a 70 percent and 90 percent improvement rate within a year of the treatment. Some patients report they feel better within a week, most within a few months, and some after an entire year.

There hasn't been enough data on why some people improve faster than others, but studies of petri-dish stem cell growth have shown increased production of stem cells. A petri dish is used to grow stem cells in a laboratory and the cells' actions in this artificial environment do not always translate into the same behavior inside a human being. Over the next decade, we will continue to discover the complexities of stem cell functions to enable us to produce specific cells for specific treatments.

Eventually, as this subject is better understood, rules and regulations will allow patients to grow their own cells prior to deployment. Our expanding knowledge will help protocols work better, but the good thing is that there has been nothing dangerous about the treatments so far. In our practice, we have primarily used adult stem cells to repair age- or trauma-related joint damage, which is the commonest type of injury we see in our practice.

There are plenty of cases of autoimmune disease that have been treated successfully with stem cells, but our practice deals primarily with patients suffering from chronic pain. We specialize in treatment programs for pain. But not all treatments are the same. Knowing where to inject for a hip or a knee condition, for example, may be pretty easy for me to do. But when it comes to something more nuanced, such as a spinal injection, there are just too many factors involved to simply make a guess based on an MRI or x-ray image.

For such complicated procedures, we use MRIs coupled with an injected radioactive dye so that the affected areas will clearly be shown on the image. This is an excellent alternative compared to the traditional MRI without contrast that will show all of the structures but not necessarily the area of injury.

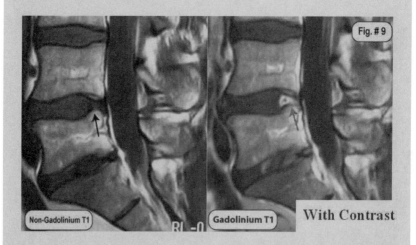

Fig. # 9

Non-Gadolinium T1

Gadolinium T1   With Contrast

Note that this MRI image shows a bright spot on the L4/5 disc, indicative of a bulge and tear in the disc.

The procedure to deliver stem cells in this area will be almost identical to an epidural injection, except that, in our case, the medication is replaced by stem cells.

SHOULDER PAIN

The shoulder is formed by the scapula, humerus, and clavicle, which make up a ball-and-socket joint. As is the case with the knee and the hip, the ends of these connecting bones are covered with articular cartilage, allowing for smooth, uninhibited movement. The shoulder forms the rotator cuff, which is composed of the supraspinatus, infaspinatus, subscapularis, and the teres minor muscles. Covering the muscles of the rotator cuff are the powerful deltoids. Torn rotator cuffs are a frequently reported cause of shoulder pain.

Complications of Surgery

1. *Problems with total shoulder replacement.* Most of the time, shoulder replacement is successful, but there are occasions when complications can arise. Complications involving rotator cuff damage are particularly troubling. This happens when the muscles of the shoulder's rotator cuff are damaged either during or shortly after the surgery.

2. *Problems with reverse total shoulder replacement.* Common complications of reverse shoulder replacement are nerve damage, dislocation, and infection. Dislocation usually involves a sudden dislocation of the socket and ball of the implant.

Common Conditions Treated with Stem Cells

The shoulder is a delicate piece of biological machinery and we usually don't realize how important it is until we can no longer use it properly. Fortunately, many of these conditions can be successfully treated with stem cells.

Here are a few of the most common conditions.

1. *Rotator cuff tears.* The rotator cuff is a combination of tendons and muscles that serve as the connective bridge between the upper arm and shoulder, facilitating a wide range of movement. Rotator cuff tears are a rather painful condition involving torn tissue, but they can be fixed with a simple injection of stem cells.

2. *Chronic impingement syndrome.* Chronic impingement syndrome involves injury to the bursae and muscles of the shoulder when it is pinched in certain positions. Many patients with this condition are given pharmaceutical drugs and a regimen of physical therapy to correct the condition, but there is now even further hope out there due to new strides in treating chronic impingement syndrome with stem cell therapy.

3. *Labral tears.* Labral tears (the labrum is the cushiony cartilage material in a joint) are usually caused by a quick twisting motion of the hip. A common symptom of this tear is a clicking sound in the shoulder when it moves through its range of motion, followed by severe, stabbing, radiating pain. Labral tears are a common problem and stem cells offer the solution.

4. *Arthritis.* Arthritis, or inflammation of the joints, can occur at any age but is most common in the elderly. Arthritis is all about inflammation, and with a quick shot of stem cells, most sufferers feel better.

Stem Cell Treatment of the Joint

1. *Injection under imaging.* Guided imaging is used to find the correct injection site and help push the stem cells to the right part of the body.

2. *Recommend physical therapy.* If the patient's condition isn't severe, walking, swimming and low-intensity aerobic exercise are good forms of physical therapy.

3. *Key areas to strengthen.* When it comes to the shoulder, the key areas you really need to strengthen are the rotator cuff and other important ligaments and muscles. Strengthening these muscles will do much to speed up the recovery process after treatment.

GERRY D.'S STORY

"I had joint pain for over twenty years. I suffered from arthritis and rotator cuff tears in my shoulders and didn't have time to be down and out with shoulder surgery. I have an air conditioning business and frequently have to work on ducting above my head and lifting items into ceilings, and I was beginning to suffer more and more at the end of the day. I considered surgery but knew my business would suffer if I couldn't be out in the field. Plus, with my deductible and coinsurance, shoulder surgery wasn't going to be cheap either.

"I wasn't scared of getting surgery, but I was concerned if it didn't work out. I was also concerned about the downtime and the lost income, which is why the stem cell treatment was a no-brainer. I was surprised at how cheap it was compared to what I had heard. Overall, I would say it was a great experience."

Gerry D., air conditioning repair, CA

JAMES'S STORY

James, a retired golf professional and total-shoulder surgery candidate, came to our office after one of his friends had had great success with stem cell therapy. When he was growing up, James was an avid athlete. He lived in an active community and enjoyed playing competitive tennis and golf until his shoulder pain became too much to bear. That is when he went to the local orthopedic center and the surgeon recommended two total-shoulder replacements because he had severe arthritic changes in both his shoulders. He even had large bone spurs that limited his ability to raise his arms above his head. But both procedures would take James away from sports for three years, which he didn't want, especially since he was in his late seventies and wasn't sure he would be able to return to his sporting activities. James was another of those who don't want to gamble on surgery. He knew that the stem cells were not going to get rid of the large bone spurs that limited his ability to perform an overarm tennis serve, but he was okay with that since surgery also wouldn't have fixed that problem. James just wanted to sleep, play tennis, golf, and perform other activities such as driving without pain, which is why he proceeded with the stem cell treatment.

James's procedure was simple: We just put into his shoulder a double dose of stem cells mixed with another product to enhance the growth and proliferation of the cells. He received light therapy on his shoulders for about a month and deep tissue work and physical therapy for about eight weeks. Golf was the first activity he was able to perform, while tennis required the full six months of cartilage growth for him to play without pain. James is another success story, and he has sent over to our clinic a few others who were suffering with rotator cuff and arthritic change in their shoulders.

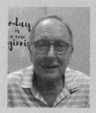

James, retired golf pro, CA—shoulder arthritis

JEFF'S STORY

Jeff sought out treatment in our office after damaging both shoulders through weight lifting. He wasn't ready to go down that surgical path, which is why he opted for a cost-effective growth factor treatment; details about this procedure will be mentioned in chapter 13.

Jeff received just one of these procedures before he was able to return to weight lifting after taking months off, resting his shoulders to heal them. He had received physical therapy, and when that didn't work, he knew he had to try something different, which is what brought him into our office. The beauty of PRP is that it is extremely cost effective and can be delivered in just one office visit.

"Four months ago, I couldn't even lift a coffee mug due to a torn Rotator cuff. After trying an experiemental Platelet Rich Plasma (PRP) shot, I'm now 99 percent! #NoSurgery!"

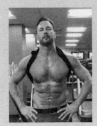

Jeff Castle, actor, CA– shoulder pain

ANKLE PAIN

The ankle presents itself as a rather inconspicuous joint—that is, until something goes wrong with it. The ankle has the big job of bearing our weight and allowing us to walk, but constant pain can make these tasks impossible. The ankle is made up of three main bones—the fibula, the tibia, and the talus—otherwise known as the two main shin bones and the heel of the foot.

Complications of Surgery

1. *Infection.* As mentioned previously in this book, just about any surgical procedure has a slight chance of infection. When infection does occur, it usually remains minor and is situated over the point of incision. If the infection spreads deeper, however, and reaches the bones themselves, the condition could become quite serious. Patients with such an infection need to receive immediate treatment.

2. *Complications with hardware.* Artificial hardware such as screws and plates placed in the ankle can cause pain and become unstable over time. Since there is little cushioning fatty tissue in the ankle, these support structures are often fixed directly on the bone. As a result, they can become painful protrusions.

3. *Nonunion/bad fusion of bones.* Edges of the fracture that are set too far apart can prevent the union of the bones and impair healing. A soft fibrous attachment may form in between the fractured edges, leading to even more complications from the bad fusion that develops.

4. *Development of pain in other joints.* Your ankle needs to have some flexibility, and when it is fused or replaced, it will never have the same mobility it once had, which often leads to more back and hip pain in the future from walking abnormally for the remainder of your life.

Common Conditions Treated with Stem Cells

1. *Ankle arthritis.* Any arthritis is painful, but ankle arthritis pain can be especially acute. Stem cells, however, are able

to reduce all inflammation once introduced with a quick, easy injection.

2. *Tendon tears.* The tendon fixed to the outside of our ankles serves to provide some stability as we walk, but if this tendon gets torn, disaster is the result. However, stem cell therapy can help to heal it

Stem Cell Treatment of the Joint

There are a few treatment options that the patient should be aware of regarding the procedure.

1. *Injection under imaging.* First, we need to determine what is causing the foot or ankle pain and where it is originating. If a tendon or ligament is causing the pain, for example, we will have to treat that tendon or ligament. Once this is determined, guided imagery can be used to direct the stem cells to the exact spot where they are needed.

2. *Recommended physical therapy.* Unfortunately, many patients do not seek out treatment for many months, or more likely, years, so most of our patients have developed balance problems and weakened muscles around the ankle joint because they have not been actively using the joint. That is why we recommend physical therapy for all of our patients. These exercises are focused on returning mobility to the ankle while adding stability to the hip, pelvis, and ankle muscles. Many people underestimate the importance of adding stability to the hip as well as improving ankle balance, but it makes a big difference to this type of patient, especially if it is a chronic condition. We don't have time to belabor this point here, but we have our patients work with

a competent rehabilitation specialist who understands this area of medicine.

3. *Key areas to strengthen.* The key areas to strengthen are the foot and the ankle itself.

"My work has taken me all over the world through extremely rough terrain, which has led to my ankle problems over the years. I was always athletic and wore excellent footwear when hiking in foreign countries, exploring new sites and discoveries, but when you twist your ankle after sliding down part of a mountain in the middle of nowhere, you are forced to just walk it off. That type of situation occurred over my career, and by the time I was getting ready for retirement, my ankles had become extremely arthritic."

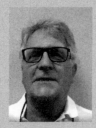

Mike, geologist, Canada

Cortisone and pain medications along with some physical therapy comprise the typical treatment for this condition, but for an active, healthy individual like Mike, this is not a good option. Healthy men live longer and ankle fusions do not work out well in the long run, which is what prompted Mike to move forward with the stem cell procedure.

The procedure itself is a simple set of injections into the ankle and into other areas that are arthritic, followed by some type of therapy to boost the growth of the stem cells. After about one month, the patient begins to work on ankle mobility exercises along with hip and ankle balance exercises. Because patients have not been actively stressing the ankle, we have to build up the balance and the strength of the bad ankle.

Patients like Mike do very well with this type of procedure, especially if the problem is caught before it reaches end-stage arthritis.

SUPPORTIVE THERAPIES

Class 4 therapeutic laser treatment, approved by the FDA in 2003, is an effective tool for decreasing pain and swelling, while dilating blood vessels to increase blood flow. Plenty of my patients have reported that the laser therapy they received at other clinics did not help them. This is because they had cold laser therapy, a lower-level laser treatment (LLLT) also called class 3 laser. LLLT uses near-infrared nonthermal lasers from five to five hundred milliwatts, with a wavelength of between six hundred and a thousand nanometers. These lasers are less powerful than a barcode scanner, so it should not surprise anyone that they are not terribly effective at increasing circulation and healing.

In contrast, class 4 laser therapy uses three watts of energy and has been shown to increase circulation in the location of use. Laser therapy has been shown to increased stem cell survival, proliferation, and homing. This means that the stem cells can better locate the damage, multiply, and survive for longer periods of time. Laser therapy also decreases cell death and results in better overall function.

PEMF Therapy

PEMF therapy (pulsed electromagnetic field) therapy has a directly positive effect on the energy balance and health of cells. Having healthy and energy-rich cells means faster and more efficient healing, not to mention better overall health. When energy is depleted, the cells' interactions are weakened, and they are vulnerable to disease. Although, we often forget this, the function of our body is based on electrically charged atoms and molecules that must interact with each other to perform every essential process in the body.

Electromagnetic energy is all around us. The earth has an electromagnetic field (EMF) that interacts with solar wind, charged particles in the solar system. This interaction protects us from a depleted ozone layer and therefore helps to safeguard us from the electromagnetic field of radiation from the sun.

Schumann resonances, electromagnetic changes, occur between the earth's surface and the lower level of the ionosphere at about forty-five to fifty kilometers above the earth's surface. These global electromagnetic resonances are generated and excited by lightning discharges near the earth's surface. These shifts in the EMF of the earth have been shown to induce health changes in living organisms, such as blood pressure changes.

Too much or too little electromagnetic charge is dangerous for all life. Human cells should, optimally, carry a charge of minus twenty to twenty-five millivolts, needing about minus fifty millivolts to replicate or build new cells. When voltage drops below minus twenty, the cell becomes vulnerable to disease. Because hydrogen atoms are positively changed, voltage is linked to pH, so a pH of 7.34 to 7.45 is best. Grounding, exercise, and drinking natural spring water are very good ways to restore the body's normal electrical charge, but the most effective way is PEMF therapy.

Low-frequency PEMFs penetrate cells while passing through the body without being absorbed or altered! When they move through the body, they stimulate electrical and chemical processes in the tissues. Therapeutic PEMFs can add balancing frequencies to the body to decrease the negative effects of EMFs.

PEMFs have been shown to:

- reduce pain, inflammation, the effects of stress on the body, and platelet adhesion;

- improve energy, blood and tissue oxygenation, circulation, sleep quality, blood pressure and cholesterol levels, the uptake of nutrients, cellular detoxification and the ability to regenerate cells;

- balance the immune system and stimulate RNA and DNA;

- accelerate repair of bone and soft tissue; and

- relax muscles.

PEMF therapy has been shown time and time again to promote healing in knee and other orthopedic injuries. As a stand-alone therapy, PEMF can reduce symptoms in patients with osteoarthritis of the knee. PEMF has also increased the regrowth of torn tendon cells, without surgery.

PEMF has been found to be synergistic with stem cells, increasing their ability to differentiate into new bone cells. Specific frequencies and duration of PEMF also increases the ability of stem cells to rebuild cartilage. Both PEMF and stem cells have powerful benefits of their own, but when used together by an experienced provider, the healing benefits can be exponential!

Healing at Home

We have many tools for helping your knee heal in my office, but some of the work must be done when you go home. As mentioned earlier in this chapter, overall health is paramount to a full recovery. This means that nutrition and other lifestyle habits alongside physical therapy are imperative for healing.

One of the biggest roadblocks to healing a weight-bearing joint such as the knee is excess weight. Too much pressure on the joint reduces space in the joint for synovial fluid and increases friction between the bones and ligaments. If our patients are not already at a healthy weight, we help them reach that goal once they leave the office. Many people think that, without exercise, this is impossible, but we're here to tell you that diet is a much more effective way to find and maintain a healthy weight.

We encourage our patients to follow a moderate ketogenic diet after treatment. This means tons of veggies, nuts, seeds, plant oils, and moderate amounts of high-quality meat and eggs. This style of eating is dense in nutrients that the body needs to properly heal. The other benefit is that by reducing carbohydrates and increasing the intake of healthy fats, our patients drop extra weight fast and enjoy the powerful anti-inflammatory benefits of balanced blood sugar. It is not uncommon for many patients to lose upward of 10 percent of their body weight in six to eight weeks after treatment.

Although most people don't know it, oftentimes they have underlying food sensitivities that cause ongoing inflammatory reactions in the body. That chronic stimulation of the immune system impedes healing, so we advise food sensitivity testing for our patients, so they can eliminate foods that disrupt healing.

Personalizing aftercare by identifying specific nutrient deficiencies in patients enhances healing. We send most patients home with tailored nutritional supplements to give their bodies an extra boost. For instance, if your body is low in vitamins C or D, your immune system and regenerative function will not be working at full capacity.

Any habit that weakens the body, such as smoking, drinking, etc., impedes healing. It's critical for our patients to take their healing seriously and do everything within their power to break habits that get in the way of their body's innate ability to repair and regenerate tissue.

Aside from healthy habits, most patients benefit from four to eight weeks of physical therapy after treatment. This is imperative for rebuilding supporting muscles and other tissues as well as increasing range of motion. Key areas to strengthen are the calf, hamstring, quads, glutes, and lower abdominals.

I can't overstate the importance of aftercare. Just last spring, Bob, a new patient, began treatment for chronic knee pain from a decades-old football injury that had progressed to arthritis and a torn meniscus. Bob was an avid golfer, but over the years, he had put on at least fifty pounds of extra weight, and between that and knee pain, he could no longer walk his favorite course. This disability made him feel he'd come to the end of life as he knew it, and he resigned to letting himself go. He said that if he could no longer walk the course with his social group a couple of times a week, or move around freely with his wife, he didn't really see the point of getting out and trying to do anything. He was depressed and becoming more sedentary and isolated each day. It's hard for people to understand how impactful a knee injury and chronic pain can be, and while it is a localized problem, it can lead to health issues throughout the body and mind.

Bob agreed to give his treatment one last shot before throwing in the towel. He underwent a stem cell injection and PEMF and laser therapy, and went home with personalized care instructions, including diet, nutrient therapy, and physical therapy. He only showed up for physical therapy, ignoring the lifestyle recommendations that had been made. When we met for a follow-up appointment, Bob made some pretty sad excuses for not following the important advice that had been given him.

But after being reminded that *all* the post-care instructions were critical for a full recovery, Bob finally listened and even convinced his wife to get on board. The next time we saw Bob was four weeks later. His weight was down by twenty pounds. His reduced inflammation was apparent in everything from a recognizable reduction in bloating to a youthful complexion that had taken the place of ruddy and blotchy skin and he could walk unhindered. You could say that Bob had a skip in his step. He said he literally could not remember a time when he felt better. He was back out with friends and could engage in all his old activities, and he gained a lot of confidence from the attention he received from members of his social circle who were impressed by how young and vibrant he felt and looked. It may have been a simple knee therapy, but the benefits were far-reaching.

Bob's experience is not uncommon for people who "buy in" and do the hard work at home. They not only get the best results from their treatment but also enjoy better all-around health. When patients ask us why they should try an alternative to pain management and surgery, we usually tell them those therapies don't work 100 percent of the time. No medical procedures do. However, the question that should be asked is—why should they not do something different? If all the other options have not fixed their problem, why would they continue them?

Try something new! Give your body the chance to heal. Each time I see a patient who was once debilitated but now walks out of my office, healthy and vibrant, I am amazed at the body's strength and resilience when given the right tools. I encourage you to trust in your body and try a new way of healing now!

Chapter 11

NEUROLOGICAL AND AUTOIMMUNE CONDITIONS

What about neurological conditions? Since stem cells can turn into nerve cells, there are cases of neurological diseases such as Parkinson's disease, strokes, and demyelinating conditions that have shown improvement. Stem cell therapy is not a panacea, nor is it a cure for these conditions, but some outcomes have been very favorable. As options go, stem cell therapy is better than surgery or the side effects of medications for these conditions, especially since it can be tried virtually risk-free.

MULTIPLE SCLEROSIS

Out of all the autoimmune disorders, multiple sclerosis (MS) is one of the worst. Multiple sclerosis originates in the killer T-cells that are able to cross the blood-brain barrier (BBB). Once across this threshold, these T-cells, which usually go after harmful foreign invaders, begin to attack the myelin sheath (outer covering of the MS patient's nerve cells). T-cells are not, normally, in abundance along the spine, yet for some reason, they become triggered to converge to that area, where they rapidly multiply.

Once there, they can wreak havoc on motor function and a wide range of movement. It is still not entirely clear what triggers the immune system to attack nerve cells, but what is abundantly clear is the kind of devastation that results. Patients suffering with MS find themselves with severe difficulty in walking, extreme muscle weakness, and fatigue, and in some cases, they may have blurry vision or even near-blindness, all due to this overabundance of unhinged T-cells.

But a batch of MSCs introduced into the patients' system is able to completely block these rogue T-cells and keep them from expanding. And this ability seems to be T-cell specific, without any additional blocking of, or interference with, the other key components of the immune system; the rest of the immune system is allowed to remain completely intact while only this one specific aspect is targeted.

This discretion stands in stark contrast to the drugs that suppress the immune system in its entirety, putting the patient at risk of worsening illness. These new studies advocating the use of stem cells have shown a possible way out of this devastating illness. When considering the future of regenerative medicine, some even feel that it wouldn't be at all too bold to say that a complete cure for multiple sclerosis could be in the cards.

When it comes to the treatment protocols for autoimmune conditions, delivery methods will vary. And over time. all providers will start to move toward one single method. To date, delivery methods include the following:

IV Delivery: Cells from birth tissue or stromal vascular fraction from fat have been used in IV therapy. The theory of this procedure is that the stem cells will be drawn to the areas of inflammation and damage. This is the most common procedure practiced in private facilities and has shown some promise.

Intrathecal Delivery: Some clinics have experimented with intrathecal deployment of stem cells; stem cells are delivered right into the spinal cord so they will make their way to the brain and pass the blood brain barrier. This is a less commonly practiced method, but it has been used in various clinics in the country.

Intranasal Delivery: This type of delivery is experimental and is promising for patients with certain types of brain disorders such a recent stroke or multiple sclerosis. By going through the nose, stem cells can be delivered directly to the brain, encouraging the development of healthy brain tissues.

TREATMENT OF PERIPHERAL NEUROPATHY

Peripheral neuropathy can be a debilitating disease affecting the nerves outside the brain and spine and leading to the abnormal functioning of the nerves. Such damage, typically, occurs with a "glove-like or stocking-like" distribution and can be wide-ranging, affecting:

- sensory nerves that detect temperature, pain, vibration, touch, among other sensations;

- motor nerves that control muscle movement; and

- autonomic nerves that control functions such as blood pressure, heart rate, digestion, and urination.

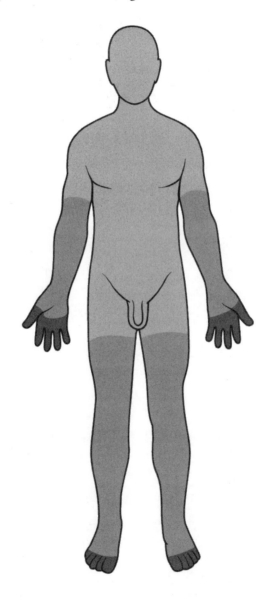

The problem with this disease is that the medications prescribed by a neurologist fall into one of the following three drug categories:

1. antiseizure: Gabapentin (Neurontin) or Lyrica

2. antidepressant: Cymbalta

3. narcotics (pain killers and anti-inflammatories): Vicodin (hydrocodone), Norco (hydrocodone-acetaminophen), Percocet, Oxycontin, Tramadol, etc.

This can be quite a problem because these drugs often become habit forming some (narcotics) of them have caused a lot of pain and suffering throughout the country. The other medications just come with many side effects, which can often be worse than the symptoms themselves, which is why many who suffer with neuropathy seek out this treatment. Neuropathy many causes, but the commonest ones we see in our office are poor circulation, age-related conditions, diabetes, and chemotherapy-induced neuropathy. Some people will develop neuropathy as a result of other conditions such as: alcoholism, HIV medications, autoimmune disease and many other causes.

The reason this is such a big deal is because the traditional treatment only focuses on the pain, which will allow you to function to a certain degree, but those medications have many side effects and can be very dangerous in the long term. To add insult to injury, none of the medications actually help the nerves heal. Typically, as this disease progresses and becomes more chronic, patients develop increasing numbness in their feet and legs.

This truly is a degenerative illness. Without the ability to feel normal pressure and receive proprioceptive feedback in the nervous system from the feet and legs, a patient's balance will be diminished. This disease, generally, affects the elderly, who also have a much higher chance of breaking a hip, wrist, or other important area when they fall. We have even had patients who have lost their driver's licenses because they caused a car accident when they stepped on the gas pedal instead of the brake pedal.

Losing a driver's license is a major blow for anyone, but for peripheral neuropathy sufferers, it can mean losing a vital means of independence, which will put more of a burden on their family and never ends well. The treatment for this condition varies, depending on the cause, but usually involves the injection of regenerative stem cells, or PRP, or other healing solutions along the damaged nerves in the feet, legs, and possibly, hands. Other treatments may involve some type of light and electrotherapy, which will improve circulation and stimulate nerve firing. There is much more to this protocol, but I wanted to give you an introductory idea of the treatment.

Lisa, a retired deputy sheriff and hard-working wife, always dreamed about retirement and traveling the world when she was older. Dreams like this kept her going throughout her career of protecting the public from dangerous criminals, but the most dangerous thing she had to face in her fifties was breast cancer. This was quite the battle for her, but she came out on top, thanks to modern medicine and a little bit of luck. Unfortunately, she developed severe nerve pain and numbness from the chemotherapy treatments.

This is not uncommon. Her oncologist told her that the symptoms would likely go away within a year, but a year and a half later, she was still suffering, still not sleeping, and still feeling burning and prickling sensations in her legs when she stood. Her balance was getting worse and worse, and eventually, she was forced to take an early retirement in her mid-fifties. Her plans to retire and travel the world changed, and she and her partner considered selling their home to get a more handicap-accessible home. They even looked at motorized scooters because she couldn't walk anymore.

They interviewed caretakers because Lisa's partner was still working and Lisa needed care for much of the day. That was when she was told about our practice, which offers a very different treatment from that offered by Lisa's neurologist. She knew that if she were going to change her future, she would have to do something very different. She decided to start our treatment, and after one visit, she was able to move to a cane. Within a couple of months, she didn't even require a cane to walk. Now it's been a few years and she has dramatically changed her life. She has lost weight because she began doing Crossfit workouts and turned into an athlete again. Her cloud of depression was lifted to reveal a sky of dreams and optimism.

We're not saying that you will respond as Lisa did, but if you don't call for a consultation you will never know.

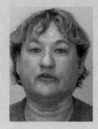

Lisa S., retired deputy sheriff

TREATMENT OF SPINAL CORD INJURIES

Of all physical traumas, injury to the spinal cord has got to be among the most traumatic. The spine is a complicated piece of biological equipment. Encased in the vertebrae are specifically separated groups of nerves. These groups are classified as cervical, thoracic, lumbar, and sacral. Spinal injury encompasses damage to any one of these segments.

Injury trauma impacts the nervous tissue encased in the vertebrae, tearing into nerve fibers and breaking apart blood vessels. The spinal cord loses a lot of blood as a result, which creates an immediate immune response in the body. Seeking to staunch the flow of blood, our immune defenses move in to rapidly form scar tissue over the injury.

Just as it does when a knee is skinned, the body quickly scabs over the torn tissue to prevent blood loss. This creates a major problem, however, because once the body produces scar tissue to cover the injury, the injured section of spinal cord is locked in place. This is how most people end up with an irreversible paralysis. It is of interest to note that, normally, after a spinal cord injury, not very many MSCs are released.

Lacking sufficient stem cells, the spine is not able to completely regenerate. It was in light of this information that researchers began to openly speculate about what MSCs might do if introduced to the site of an injured spine. Due to this interest, several clinical trials and studies were created in which spinal injury patients had MSCs introduced into their system so that tissues could be regenerated.

After the completion of several studies of therapy that used allogenic umbilical cord stem cells, it was discovered that routine treatment, generally, improved the patient's condition. In 2008, it was discovered that the severed spines of laboratory mice grew back together once they had human MSCs introduced to the injury site. What would have been a permanent disability was cured rapidly.

All of these success stories in early research have led to what clinical researchers refer to as clinical translation. This means that knowledge in the field is now substantial enough for clinicians to work on ways to translate their efforts in the laboratory to real-world medical treatments. All of these clinical trials could very well lead to a cure in the very near future.

STEM CELLS FOR THE TREATMENT OF THE AUTISTIC MIND

There has been much talk in recent years of the autism spectrum and just who might be designated to fall within those parameters. As the number of diagnoses of disorders ranging from severely disabling autism to highly dysfunctional Asperger's syndrome continues to grow, we can only wonder where it will all end—and if there will ever be a cure in sight. Most clinicians are currently focusing on how to manage behavior. Very few have considered there might actually be a cure. But the powerful realm of the stem cell just might hold that possibility.

Even though autism is not classified as an autoimmune disorder, recent research has indicated that autism may very well be connected to the immune system in ways that we have yet to fully understand. There have been several indications that those who fall into the autistic spectrum are prone to severe bouts of inflammation. Blood work of autistic patients has indicated that those with autism have large quantities of chemokines, which produce chronic inflammation.

Not only that but these same patients also often have abnormally high levels of autoantibodies, and many are found to suffer from autoimmune difficulties when it comes to digestion, with many presenting symptoms akin to those of Crohn's disease. It is estimated that roughly 20 percent of all autism patients suffer from chronic inflammation of their GI tract. At first glance, many might wonder just how problems in in the intestines can translate into problems in the brain. But the causal connection between good gut health and healthy brain chemistry is well established.

According to the experts, there is, literally, a second brain of nerves in your gut, which they like to call the enteric nervous system (ENS). This special bundle of nerves consists of a hundred million nerve cells and stretches from all the way from your esophagus to your stomach and down to your rectum. The primary job of your ENS is to help regulate digestion, but studies have shown that it also plays a role in the facilitation of emotional shifts.

In that case, *gut feeling* and *butterflies in the stomach* might be real phenomena connected to the communication between the pseudo-brain of your stomach and the brain locked inside the head. So, what does all this mean for autism and the future of regenerative medicine? It is believed that the chronically inflamed condition of the autistic gut just might be having a very real physical impact on the autistic brain. Research has clearly indicated that those with autism suffer from neuroinflammation.

According to this theory, routine treatments with stem cells, which act to subdue inflammation, could very well bring down this neuroinflammation and thereby reduce—and possibly even cure—autism. So far, those who have been given such treatments have shown a marked improvement in their ability to control their emotions and in the quality of their intellect, and they have also improved their understanding of nonverbal cues. If the trend continues, autism, with all its hallmark traits, may, eventually, be eliminated.

LUPUS

Lupus is a terrible illness that affects millions every year. The disease mostly affects women, but it has been known to strike men as well. As with any other autoimmune disease, lupus is caused by an immune response of the body that impels it to attack its own healthy tissue.

RHEUMATOID ARTHRITIS

This disorder is quite common, producing severe inflammation of the joints. About two hundred thousand new cases of rheumatoid arthritis (RA) are estimated to develop every single year. It is commonly believed to be incurable, but stem cell therapy is now promising to change that.

LAURA'S STORY

"I suffered with rheumatoid arthritis for over twenty-five years and developed chronic fatigue and chronic joint pain as a result of the disease. I have tried a number of medications that the rheumatologist prescribed, but many of them are harsh on your kidneys, liver, and immune system. I have been faithful with acupuncture, chiropractic, and physical therapy over the years. I have changed my diet and everything seemed to help. Feeling sorry for myself wasn't an option, and even though I woke up in pain, and had to drag myself to exercise classes and running errands, all I wanted to do was stay in bed. I wouldn't allow myself to do this, but when I heard about stem cell therapy I researched it diligently. I came to this center to receive treatment, and I was thankful that I went forward with this treatment. My family doctor didn't think I should do it, but I had nothing to lose and everything to gain.

"The treatment itself was a simple IV infusion of stem cells into my body, and I felt some changes in the first month, but after about four to five months, I realized I was waking up without pain and didn't feel tired anymore. I could exercise three days in a row and didn't suffer the next day anymore. I understand that the treatment doesn't cure my RA, but it really helps, and I would be more than happy to do this treatment every year or two if it improves my quality of life.

If you are even thinking about this treatment—don't! Just make it happen, because it has literally changed my life. I haven't felt like this for over twenty-five years.

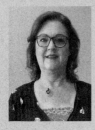

—*Laura A., home maker, WA*

PSORIATIC ARTHRITIS

Psoriatic arthritis creates a wide range of detrimental conditions in those who suffer from this disorder including brittle nails and rough, reddish spots that cover the skin. Psoriatic arthritis is a classic autoimmune disease in which the body is triggered to create an inflammatory response against an intruder that does not exist. Once triggered, the body begins to attack itself, resulting in the inflamed scales of skin so readily recognizable with psoriasis.

JACKIE'S STORY

"I was a tomboy when I was younger, always climbing trees and running around with the boys growing up. One time, I fell out of a tree when I was a kid and landed right on my rear end, and I believe that is what started most of my problems. As a result of this, I developed a lot of arthritis in my lower back, pelvis, and right hip joint, and to add insult to injury, I developed psoriatic arthritis in my adult life. Over the years, I tried to manage this pain with medications and injections and was 100 percent positive I didn't want to get surgery for this condition. I didn't know how much pain was from my psoriatic arthritis, because I hurt all over, but I definitely hurt more in my lower back and hip.

"Eventually, I got to a point where the nonsurgical treatments were not working anymore, and I wasn't ready for surgery. I knew my insurance would cover the surgeries, but something about me wasn't comfortable with back and hip surgery, which is why I decided I would try stem cell therapy. I had seen the doctors who offer this therapy and was very comfortable with their clinical competence, and when they told me I was a candidate, my husband and I decided to go forward with the treatment.

"The treatment was not much different from the injections I had received in the past. They harvested the stem cells from my own body and injected them into my hip and spine and provided IV therapy to help my psoriatic arthritis.

"I wasn't sure if it was going to work because I didn't feel much for about two to three months, but within six months, I was pain-free, and my fingers didn't hurt anymore because my psoriatic arthritis seemed to go into remission. I don't know if this is going to be the solution for psoriatic arthritis, but I think it should be. The medications my doctor wanted to put me on for my psoriatic arthritis had way too many side effects and the idea of getting cancer or major infections from those medications wasn't something I was willing to risk.

"Stem cells worked for me and they will work for you. If you suffer with psoriatic arthritis or any other disease, I highly suggest you try this treatment out."

—Jackie, retired advertising executive, CA

TREATMENT FOR DIABETICS

Given the rates at which people are succumbing to the disease, diabetes is nothing short of a modern-day scourge. And this is especially the case in the United States where it is estimated that roughly 29 million Americans suffer from the illness, making up a whopping 9 percent of the populace. And this only accounts for those with full-blown diabetes, since an even larger proportion of the population make up the count of those with symptoms of prediabetes.

The fault in the diabetes stars lies in a disruption of insulin. Both type 1 and type 2 diabetes result from the body's failure to properly use its own insulin. The pancreas of type 1 diabetics fails to produce substantial amounts of insulin, while the tissue of type 2 diabetics can no longer effectively respond to insulin and has become insulin resistant, leading to dangerously high levels of blood sugar. A potential cure has been proposed for type 1 diabetics through the use of stem cells as regenerative medicine.

It is believed that further efforts in this direction will lead to the conclusion that type 1 diabetes is an autoimmune disorder that can be cured through stem cell therapy's ability to help the pancreas to regain the ability to produce insulin. The stem cells serve to reeducate the lagging production centers of the pancreas, allowing more insulin to be produced and resulting in a healthier level of blood sugar.

Regarding type 2 diabetes, studies have shown that both MSCs and adipose-derived stem cells can help to facilitate the growth of blood vessels and encourage the production of pancreatic transcription factors and vascular growth factors, which will serve to restore proper function of insulin in the body. The future of regenerative medicine as an effective therapy for diabetics looks good.

REGENERATION OF VITAL ORGANS

It may sound like fantasy to some, but the concept of growing organs from scratch may very well become a reality. And many strides in that direction have already been made. Back in 2016, for example, a group of scientists at Harvard Medical School and Massachusetts General Hospital were able to take skin cells and transform them into pluripotent stem cells. These "induced pluripotent stem cells" as they are known were first discovered/manufactured in 2006, when regular cells taken from mice were successfully reprogrammed into embryonic stem cells. This bit of cellular engineering is accomplished through the introduction of a manipulated virus carrying genetic material that forces the cell into an embryonic state.

Now fast-forward ten years, and in 2016 we already had a handful of researchers able to induce human skin cells into becoming stem cells and grow an entire heart from the material. So far, the only real hindrance to furthering these efforts is that scientists have had a hard time growing these tissues outside the strictly controlled conditions of the laboratory. Tissue growth can, currently, only be achieved on preconstructed artificial frameworks.

In other words, there are still many complications to be worked out when it comes to implanting an artificially developed organ into the complex environment of a physical body cavity. But there is hope that, one day, a vital organ, such as the heart, can be implanted in a patient, take root, and grow there without problems.

And speaking of the future, potential breakthroughs may be in store for other diseases such as:

- Alzheimer's,

- COPD,

- congestive heart failure,

- dementia,

- kidney failure, and

- many more.

The future looks bright for stem cell treatment of conditions such as the ones presented in this chapter. But we have to remember that these conditions have not been tested to the same extent imposed on some of the others we mentioned earlier. I'm sure, over the next few decades, protocols will be developed that will produce better outcomes for some of these difficult-to-treat conditions.

For example, there are promising outcomes related to brain damage and dementia in humans who have suffered multiple concussions. Once a trial moves to human use, it is deemed safe and can yield immediate results, compared to its much humbler and slower-paced beginning in petri dish and rat studies. This exciting new field of medicine is advancing all the time. And who knows whether, within a couple of years of this book's publication, there will be another breakthrough, and we will have to write a new edition.

But as of writing this edition of our book, stem cell therapy is far from being a perfect science. We still have much to learn, and we invite you to learn it with us. In the next few chapters we will be sharing more information about growth factors, cosmetic procedures, and sexual dysfunction treatment. So stay tuned.

Chapter 12

NEW BREAKTHROUGHS IN REGENERATIVE MEDICINE THROUGH PRP

Another growth factor treatment is PRP, a nonsurgical treatment for soft-tissue injuries and joint pain. It has been performed for well over a decade. PRP stimulates the body's natural healing forces, which is an excellent way of getting the body to work in favor of the patient rather than in opposition to the patient.

Often, a patient using PRP will be able to avoid more invasive procedures such as surgery. If surgery is not an option, or the patient simply desires a less invasive procedure, PRP is a viable option with less risk and a shorter recovery time, in many cases. Chronic soft tissue injuries can be treated with PRP as an alternative to steroids. The beauty of PRP is that it has the ability to offer these alternatives in a safe and convenient package.

WHAT IS PRP?

PRP is a substance made from the patient's own blood to trigger healing. The ability to harness the power of your own body and the blood it contains to heal yourself is a definite bonus. PRP therapy is a relatively simple, nonsurgical treatment for joint injuries and arthritis. It merges cutting-edge technology with the body's natural ability to heal itself.

It is also perfectly typed and cross-matched to your body because it comes from your own body. The PRP fluid is a concentration of platelets that can jump-start healing. Platelets contain packets of growth hormones and cytokines that tell the tissues to increase rebuilding in order to enhance healing. When PRP is injected into the damaged area, it stimulates a mild inflammatory response, which triggers a healing cascade of restored blood flow, new cell growth, and tissue regeneration. When patients select PRP therapy over more invasive surgical procedures, they reap the benefits of a safer, more effective procedure that allows faster healing.

WHERE DOES PRP COME FROM?

Under sterile conditions, a sample of blood is taken from a vein in the patient's arm. The blood is placed in a centrifuge, which is a device that spins the blood down to distinct layers, based on density. This helps to separate the blood cells from the plasma and allows a concentration of the platelets. The layers can then be extracted and harvested for use. This purified sample of platelets increases the volume of healing growth factors to approximately six to eight times greater than normal.

It's simple techniques like this that make these types of regenerative procedures so effective and efficient. The preparation takes as little as fifteen minutes. The finished PRP product is then available for injection into the injured joint or tendon under ultrasound guidance. Because PRP is prepared from the patient's own blood, there is no risk of rejection or disease transmission.

In fact, PRP contains a high concentration of white blood cells, which helps to fight infection. So in contrast to the risk of infection inherent in surgery, PRP decreases the chance of infection, which is another great reason to try PRP therapy.

WHAT ARE THE POTENTIAL BENEFITS?

PRP therapy enhances the body's healing potential. It has often proven to be an effective and natural alternative to steroid injections. Patients can see a significant improvement in their symptoms as well as a return of function, which may eliminate the need for more aggressive treatments such as long-term medication or surgery.

WHAT CAN I EXPECT DURING MY TREATMENT AT YOUR OFFICE?

We will ask about your medical history and give you a brief exam to determine whether you are a good candidate for PRP therapy. If so, a sample of your blood will be drawn and the PRP prepared. We will examine the area to be treated, sterilize it, and apply an anesthetic. Typically, using ultrasound guidance, the PRP will be gently injected into the injured area and joint support tissues.

After your treatment, you will stay in our office for a thirty-minute observation period. At checkout, you will schedule a follow-up appointment and we will review discharge instructions to ensure you remain safe, comfortable, and healthy. The treatment may be repeated once or twice over a six- to sixteen-week period.

WHAT CAN I EXPECT AFTER THE PRP THERAPY?

You may have mild to moderate discomfort, which may last up to a week. There may be a temporary worsening of symptoms due to the stimulation of the inflammatory response, which is necessary for healing. Your doctor will instruct you in the use of ice, elevation, reduced activity, and analgesic medications for comfort while the PRP is initiating healing. Additionally, physical therapy or a therapeutic exercise program will be prescribed to accelerate your recovery.

WHAT SHOULD I DO WHEN I GET HOME FOLLOWING THE PROCEDURE?

Because PRP releases growth factors, it is important to not disturb the area of injection for at least forty-eight hours. We ask that you refrain from activities other than necessary walking or driving in order to receive the maximum benefit of the PRP growth factor stimulation. It is helpful if you can be sedentary for forty-eight hours and refrain from any vigorous activity for up to two weeks following the procedure.

WHAT MEDICATIONS CAN I TAKE?

Please do not take any anti-inflammatory medications such as Ibuprofen, Aleve, Motrin, and aspirin. You may take Tylenol or you may be prescribed an appropriate analgesic if necessary. If you are on a daily dose of eighty-one milligrams of aspirin for cardiovascular reasons, please do not take it within the first forty-eight hours.

PRP therapy is a very effective non-stem-cell therapy that still allows patients to avoid the use of invasive surgical procedures, and the pros of this approach far outweigh the cons.

PRP is a great alternative to try for mild to moderate degenerative conditions because of its low cost compared to all of the other options I mentioned earlier. There are no stem cells in this protocol, but the blood is fairly simple to process. It is autologously drawn (your own cells are drawn) so there is no chance of your body rejecting it, and we use an airless system, which virtually eliminates any chance of an infection. One factor we have to consider regarding PRP therapy is the patient's health, because growth factors in the blood decrease with age. The level of growth factors is also affected by the state of the patient's health, which is something to consider when comparing this therapy to amnion injections. Amniotic fluid has significantly more healing properties than PRP, but it costs more than double the price of PRP. There are many things to consider when contemplating whether surgery or stem cell treatment or something else is the best option.

Factors such as cost, safety, effectiveness, and recovery time should all be considered to ensure that the most appropriate decision is reached. Sometimes surgery can be avoided entirely, and the results of nonsurgical interventions are becoming increasingly favorable as modern science provides techniques that are increasingly more effective.

EXOSOME THERAPY

Our body ceases to amaze us, and one tiny little discovery almost thirty years ago was about harnessing the power of tiny little vesicles called exosomes. Exosomes are present in almost all bodily fluid and consist of little vesicles (little even by microscopic standards) that facilitate the transference of RNA, DNA, and protein from cell to cell. By means of such transference, exosomes control the functionality of surrounding cells. In the cellular world, exosomes know exactly who needs what and how to get them what they need.

You can think of exosomes as being an additional conductor in your physiological orchestra or the dispatcher for a large construction company. Stem cells are the construction workers that rely on cell signals they receive from the site of injury, but exosomes actively recruit other types of regenerative cells to the site of injury and use cell signaling to speed up the healing process. The exosome approach to therapy is far-reaching, from packaging therapeutic agents to driving immune responses in fields ranging from oncology to regenerative medicine.

Exosomes are basically the janitors of cellular debris. They work hard to clean up cell waste, but that's not all—exosomes also serve as crucial messengers, sending signals from one area to another. You see, the tiny little vesicles in the cellular membrane that exosomes consist of are loaded with lipids, protein, and other cellular ingredients crucial for proper physiological function. It is for this reason that exosomes are being used to treat autoimmune disorders in which the body's natural cellular communication is disrupted.

To put it quite simply, our cells like to speak to each other, and the silent treatment that degenerative disorders engender is not good for anyone. The introduction of exosomes, however, can help facilitate and restore this vital line of communication between cells. Due to their small size, they can even cross over the "blood brain barrier," bypassing the "checkpoints" and sending direct signals to the brain. This is tremendously important for those suffering from the aftermath of a stroke.

The small tubular shaped exosome may be like a needle in a physiological haystack, but it is able to go where other molecular structures fear to tread. The fact that exosomes provide another neural pathway to the brain when other options for the stroke patient are off the table is nothing short of revolutionary. In fact, exosome therapy for stroke patients has become a leading form of treatment.

Exosomes have also proven to be quite useful when it comes to the treatment of those who suffer from asthma. Asthma, although a common ailment, is a chronic form of respiratory discomfort for those that suffer from it. And if conditions worsen enough, asthma can even be life threatening. Exosomes have proven quite beneficial, however, in communicating to the tissues of the inflamed bronchial tubes of asthmatics.

What does that mean in plain English? Exosomes are able to get the lungs to loosen up, and relieve the chronic tightness in the chest so familiar to asthma patients. Exosomes can be the message runner, telling tissues to lighten up so inflamed airways can open once again. As this crucial piece of the physiological puzzle, exosomes can really do wonders. Exosomes are able to effectively pass messages to the central nervous system giving it the all clear to tone down inflammation.

Regular treatment from exosomes promises to better regulate this function in asthma suffers. So, for those whose inhaler just doesn't seem to cut it, exosome therapy promises an exciting alternative. These are just a few examples of how exosome therapy could be (pun only slightly intended) just what the doctor ordered!

Chapter 13

COSMETIC USES FOR REGENERATIVE MEDICINE

Besides boosting our immunity and increasing the speed of healing, PRP therapy can even make us look better!

Yes, it's true. There are many trials underway investigating potential cosmetic uses for PRP therapy. Along with PRP therapy, mesotherapy is another new frontier in cosmetic regenerative medicine in which powerful medical extracts are injected right into the skin. If you are looking for a viable alternative to plastic surgery, check out the procedures discussed in this chapter.

PRP INJECTIONS IN COSMETICS

As mentioned elsewhere in this book, PRP injections have been successfully used to treat a wide variety of ailments from sports injuries to urinary incontinence and sexual dysfunction. But what possible role can PRP injections play in the world of cosmetics? Well, just as platelet-rich plasma can speed up the healing process in other weak and damaged tissue in the body, it can also work to rejuvenate and restore faltering tissue of the skin, hair, hair, and nails.

Wrinkles, brittle nails, and frayed hair are due to the depletion of collagen. Collagen is the binding superglue of our bodies, holding everything in place. As collagen begins to diminish, soft tissue such as skin, for example, begins to droop and sag, becoming much less firm than it was in the past. An injection of PRP can get your collagen back in working order.

PRP FOR THE HAIR

It is said that 70 percent of all people on the planet will come to experience some form of hair loss or thinning during the course of their life. With such regularity of this occurrence, you would think there would be more demand for a cure than there already is. But instead of clamoring for solutions, most simply accept their hair loss and suffer in silence. PRP offers a way out of the doldrums of diminishing hair, however, through the use of injections of platelet-rich plasma.

Using scalp-specific growth factors, PRP treatments can work to stimulate the hair follicles, thereby encouraging new hair growth. If a patient has a thinning or bald patch of hair, PRP treatment can revitalize the site, allowing the hair to grow properly once again. Platelets are the body's answer to inflammation. As soon as a highly-concentrated number of platelets arrive on the scene, they automatically begin the process of restoring damaged tissue. When the scalp and damaged hair follicles are targeted with this PRP formula, hair will begin to grow again.

THE VAMPIRE FACELIFT

Made famous by the likes of Kim Kardashian, the vampire facelift is a noninvasive procedure that involves the delivery of highly concentrated PRP fibrin matrix, coupled with additional growth factors from the blood and a potent hyaluronic acid dermal filler applied directly to the face. This procedure has shown much promise in combating wrinkles and adding volume and quality to the skin. That said, the vampire facelift may not work in quite the same way on everyone and tends to vary in efficiency depending on the severity of deterioration.

In other words, if someone's face is completely full of wrinkles, the vampire facelift may not provide the most immediate results. For those with more severe skin damage, plastic surgery may be the better option. But for those with mild to moderate deterioration of the skin, the vampire facelift can certainly do wonders. The vampire facelift is especially good at filling in spaces that have lost their natural volume. It can do this with skin, muscle, fat, and even bone.

Those with depleted stores of tissue in these areas often have sunken eyes, faltering eyelids, a saggy neck, and skin with a greyish hue. The vampire facelift can help fill in those sunken eyes and bring a rosy glow back to the surface of the skin. The rosy glow in particular is brought about by the growth of new blood vessels, which bring more blood to the face, resulting in a healthy flushed appearance.

Possible side effects of treatment include:

- feelings of intense pressure at the injection site,

- lingering redness or swelling on the face,

- prevalence of bruising or tenderness,

- prolonged numbing or tingling sensation, and

- possible exacerbation of symptoms from alcohol consumption.

Postoperative recommendations are as follows:

- Patients should restrict physical contact with the injection site in the first few hours after the procedure.

- If possible, patients should sleep flat on their back, with their head slightly raised for several days after the procedure.

- Patients should stay out of direct sunlight for a few days after the procedure.

- Facials should be avoided for a couple of weeks after the procedure.

- The face should not be washed for the first few hours after the procedure.

Although Kim Kardashian's famous results may have been a little less than stellar, all in all, the vampire facelift has produced some rather promising results. After the procedure, the treatment remains in full effect for the next few months, and the beneficial regeneration of the can last to a year, after which the wrinkles and sagging may return.

Before   **After**

Notice the bags and the fine lines and see how they disappear
after treatment.

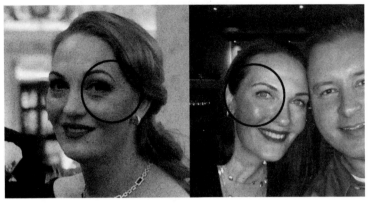

MESOTHERAPY FOR THE HAIR

Many people suffer from baldness or thinning hair, but few know
how to combat the problem. Mesotherapy offers a unique way
forward. Through the process of mesotherapy, the scalp is injected
with special nutrient boosters that are specifically geared toward the
nourishment and hydration of the scalp. This nutritional boost will
jumpstart the cellular metabolism of the scalp, kick-starting the new
growth of hair. Improved blood flow will also serve to strengthen the
hair follicles so that much more voluminous hair can form rapidly.

Mesotherapy is usually conducted with the use of microinjec-
tions that are inserted just under the surface of the scalp. These needles
work to create several microperforations, injecting the nutrients into
the skin and promoting the healing response of the body. As a result,
the powerful connective tissues of collagen and elastin move in to
restore the scalp to its former pristine glory. When it comes to finding
effective new cosmetic use for regenerative medicine, mesotherapy
has gone above and beyond expectations, as have all the methods
described in this chapter.

Chapter 14

SEXUAL DYSFUNCTION AND HOW PRP CAN HELP

It's not any easy subject to discuss, but sexual dysfunction is a common problem and it's not one that has to be answered by way of over-the-counter prescriptions. In this chapter, we will discuss the many forms of regenerative medicine that can be utilized in order to safeguard their users from all manner of sexual dysfunction.

ERECTILE DYSFUNCTION: AN EMBARRASSING YET COMMON PROBLEM

Most men are afraid to talk about it, but according to the latest statistics, up to 40 percent of men age forty and up have trouble with erectile dysfunction (ED). According to the latest research, this number is increasing. In fact, a recent study conducted by the

Journal of Sexual Medicine has compiled some rather startling data to indicate that ED is becoming much more prevalent among younger generations.

So never mind all the guys in their forties, because there are now plenty of men under the age of forty who are having much the same problem. So, what is causing all of this difficulty? Well, if you thought that your problems in the bedroom were all in your mind, you just might be right, because anxiety has been cited as the leading cause of erectile dysfunction. Another factor cited in this sudden climb in ED in the younger generation is the increasingly unhealthy diet that many consume.

A diet loaded with sugar and carbohydrates is not only bad for the figure but also harms the heart and blood flow, thereby wrecking the ability of blood to properly flow down to the penis to produce an erection. A poor diet can also mess up the body's hormone balance, adversely affecting the production of testosterone. This is due to an overabundance of certain testosterone-suppressing chemical compounds that can be found in some overly processed foods.

Drugs and alcohol are other common causes of ED induced by a chemical imbalance. Drinking excessive amounts of alcohol can alter hormones. The same goes for certain drugs, especially narcotics. Right now, America is in the middle of an opioid epidemic. Along with all the other problems that this epidemic has wrought, it has been widely established that this kind of heavy narcotic, pain-relieving drug also has a devastating effect on testosterone.

However, the number-one reason for the current problem of erectile dysfunction is believed to be the sedentary life most people lead. This lack of mobility decreases the heart's ability to pump blood, which can greatly reduce the body's ability to produce and sustain an erection. ED is more common than you might think, so let's go ahead and get over the embarrassment and, instead, learn how we can use regenerative medicine to do something about it.

HOW THE P-SHOT CAN HELP YOUR ED

Ever heard of the P-shot? Probably not, but if you had, you would know it has tremendous potential to treat erectile dysfunction. The P-shot utilizes PRP. Injected directly into the penis, PRP can restore blocked blood flow to the penis and in doing so, greatly increases a man's ability to have frequent, sustained erections. And this dose of PRP is completely safe because it is autologously delivered.

PRP is a natural healer, laden with tissue-repairing growth factors and can be used to promote health and wellness in a wide variety of ways. In order to benefit from this procedure, the patient simply needs to undergo a basic blood draw, which is then centrifuged to extract the PRP. For most men, injecting the PRP directly into the penis is the most challenging part of the experience, but there really is nothing to fear. As squeamish as the concept might make you feel, the injection site is thoroughly numbed beforehand to eliminate any pain. The entire session takes less than thirty minutes, and once it is carried out, the patient will experience an almost immediate difference as proper blood flow is restored to the penile tissue.

FEMALE SEXUAL DYSFUNCTION AND URINARY STRESS INCONTINENCE

It isn't only men who face dysfunction in the bedroom. Women can suffer many difficulties of their own, many of which are linked to urinary stress incontinence (the inability of the bladder to hold urine due to external stressors). In many cases, something as simple as a sneeze can bring about leakage, let alone anything as fundamentally invasive as sexual intercourse. In women, incidences of urinary stress incontinence begin to markedly increase between the ages of forty and sixty. And stress on a woman's urinary system has a direct impact on her reproductive system since the vagina, vulva, bladder, and urethra are all physically close to each other. In fact, the proximity of these organs can lead to many complications. For example, the rigors of childbirth can alter the position of these internal organs, which may cause additional pressure on the bladder and lead to urinary stress incontinence. Surgery such as a hysterectomy can also substantially interfere with the stability of the female urinary system, causing sexual dysfunction.

Hysterectomies are impactful because the uterus is one of the main pillars supporting the bladder and other organs. Removing it can put a woman at risk of an internal prolapse of the bladder (the bladder moves from its normal position and pushes against the walls of other organs such as the vagina and rectum). Women suffering from this condition can have severe urinary stress incontinence and accompanying sexual dysfunction.

HOW THE O-SHOT CAN HELP

The O-shot (or, as its other eye-catching moniker screams at us, the orgasm shot), is similar to the P-shot in that it contains a heavy dose of PRP. In the case of women, the targets of this PRP cocktail are the clitoris and the upper vagina, two extremely sensitive erogenous zones. Immediately before the procedure, patients are instructed to apply a topical anesthetic to the vaginal tissue slated for injection.

It is while this part of the body is growing numb that the attending physician takes a small blood sample, drawn directly from the patient's arm and centrifuged to produce the O-shot. The patient is given another injection of anesthetic before the O-shot is directly injected into the vaginal tissue. These platelets then get to work immediately, encouraging the growth of essential new tissue, such as elastin, a stretchy connective tissue.

Once the procedure has been carried out, patients are able to go home of their own accord on the very same day. The only caution given is that sexual intercourse must be avoided for the next few days. The O-shot has demonstrated an ability to treat disorders such as female sexual arousal disorder, hypoactive sexual desire disorder, female orgasmic disorder, and vaginal dryness, as well as providing much needed relief to bouts of urinary stress incontinence.

Here are a few direct benefits of the O-shot that patients have reported:

- an improved libido;

- a tighter vagina;

- a more easily aroused clitoris;

- improved skin tone of external genitals;

- increased incidence of orgasm, and a more powerful orgasm;

- increase in the production of vaginal lubricant; and

- reduced incidence of discomfort during intimacy.

Sexual dysfunction is not something to hide or be embarrassed about, and as you can see from this chapter, there are several regenerative solutions for whatever problem someone may be facing. As the O-shot and P-shot demonstrate, PRP therapies are extremely effective in restoring sexual function.

Chapter 15

BANKING YOUR STEM CELLS FOR THE FUTURE

Imagine that you are playing a game of tennis when you hear a pop in your knee and find out that you have torn a tendon, or imagine that you have a chronic condition such as rheumatoid arthritis that eats away at your body, or imagine that you have had a stroke and damaged your brain. Imagine being able to treat all of these conditions with your very own cells made from your own DNA. Your body makes trillions of stem cells over time, but as you age, these cells are replenished at a slower rate, and eventually, parts of your body start to break down. This can lead to organ failure, tissue failure, joint failure, or even failure of your nerves, such as those in your brain. As this book has discussed, many cases of brain injury have been successfully treated with stem cell therapy when carried out *within a proximate window of time*. But how do we protect ourselves from unforeseen health problems in our later years when our cells no longer function as well as they did when we were younger and we need immediate access to the healing power of healthy cells? The answer is bioinsurance.

CELL BANKING AND STORAGE

Bioinsurance is a growing field in which a facility will store your cells for potential treatment of future chronic diseases. The cells are banked before they are needed, just as car insurance provides protection against the possibility of a future accident.

In many ways, stem cells are only as good as their storage. If they are not stored properly, they will rapidly deteriorate. To be viable, they must be stored properly. That said, let's take a brief look at stem cell storage.

How Are Stem Cells Stored?

All donated cell-stem-related biological material is placed in a tissue bank to be screened and processed, after which it is held in state of cryopreservation until needed. This means it is frozen to preserve the tissue without destroying the cells. The material is kept frozen at about minus 200° Celsius (which is 328° below zero in Fahrenheit) in an automated, microprocessor-controlled cell freezer. These containment units are full of liquid nitrogen, or liquid nitrogen vapor, which continuously regulates the temperature. Stored at these extreme temperatures, the stem cells can remain in a permanent state of viability almost indefinitely.

Benefits of Stem Cell Banking

In case you haven't heard the news, health insurance is quite a big deal at the moment. But navigating through the murky waters of health insurance can be a rather difficult experience, and the complication only increases when stem cell banking is involved. The following are some of the benefits of cell banking:

- Biological material that matches that of the patient is readily available for future treatments.

- The cell bank offers a potential treatment resource in the event of the development of cancer.

- Stored cells could be used if immune therapy were needed in the future.

- The cell bank is a treatment resource for the potential depletion of bone marrow.

- Possible future blood disorders could be treated with stored cells.

- The stored cells provide a treatment option for the potential development of osteoporosis.

Banking Saves Time and Money on Future Procedures

It used to be that stem cell therapy was a luxury that only the superrich could afford. In recent years, things have changed quite a bit. Stem cell therapy is now more affordable, and the best way to save time and money on future procedures is through stem cell banking. All of us have physical bodies that deteriorate over time. Sooner or later, most of us will have to go to the hospital for a costly medical procedure. It is for that reason that, no matter what our future malady may be, having a reliable bank of stem cells could prove critical to our recovery.

Who Should Consider Cell Banking?

Eligibility for cell banking depends on the individual's specific circumstances and would be determined by a specialist in stem cell therapy.

REGENERATIVE MEDICINE TO REVERSE EFFECTS OF AGE

No matter how old we are, we would all like to look our best, right? Yet, as the clock ticks on, we all begin to show signs of wear and tear. Regenerative medicine holds out the hope that, one day, many of the effects of aging can be greatly slowed down, if not reversed completely. As author, scientist, and avid regenerative medicine enthusiast Dr. Neil Riordan recently observed, much of the aging process is due to a body whose healing capacity has become overextended with time.

We all come into this world with a limited supply of stem cells, which declines with time. However, according to Riordan, some people are born with more of this ready-made supply than others. In addition, those who have suffered one or more traumatic injuries will end up with a much more depleted bank of stem cells, since these cells have already been massively expended during the healing process.

Those who have a larger balance of these stem cells near the end of their life are the ones who age more slowly. These are the folks who are fifty-five years old yet look more like thirty-five. Many attribute this slowed-down rate of aging to the high quality and quantity of the remaining stem cells these youthful individuals possess. So, wouldn't it stand to reason that those who age more rapidly due to a lack of stem cells could benefit from stem cell injections?

Many regenerative medicine specialists are actively pursuing this logic. And as the latest clinical trials reported in *The Journals of Gerontology* indicate, a steady dose of MSCs can indeed work wonders. The first such study was done with fifteen elderly and frail subjects, who each received one shot of MSCs that had been donated from the bone marrow of younger donors.

Infused with this fresh batch of stem cells, the elderly test subjects almost immediately showed improvements in energy, vigor, vitality, and overall health. And this transformation is, apparently, much more than skin deep. Several subjects who had undergone these trials were found to have telomeres that had increased in length.

Telomeres are the protective markers found at each end of a chromosome, and they shorten as we age. The fact that these telomeres reverse course and lengthen after patients have been given fresh stem cells would seem to indicate that regenerative medicine can reverse the effects of age! This is all the more reason to look to the future and continue to keep those powerful, regenerative cells on ice! The stem cells you harvested in your younger years could provide the means of reinvigorating you in your later years by rejuvenating your aging telomeres!

Conclusion

THE RIGHT TO TRY AND THE RIGHT TO REGENERATE

The debate about regenerative medicine came into the spotlight over the recent right-to-try legislation passed by the US Congress. This federal act is intended to provide terminally ill patients across the USA with access to experimental drugs and clinical trials—including regenerative medicine—that have not yet been officially approved by the FDA. The days of stem cell tourism, when patients suffering from degenerative illness had to travel thousands of miles abroad to receive treatment, are over.

Of course, the passage of the Congressional bill did not come without controversy. While many hail the federal Right to Try Act of 2017 as a progressive window of opportunity, many oppose it on the grounds that the treatments may not be effective or even detrimental to the health of patients, thereby giving them false hope.

If this book is any testament, we have seen that the limits of medicine are not static. What was impossible yesterday may very well be possible tomorrow. And just as the eager proponents of right-to-try legislation have demonstrated, there are more than enough people ready to push that medical envelope even further. If you listen carefully, you can clearly hear the cry of these intrepid souls for the right to try, and the right to regenerate. Thank you for reading.

ONE FINAL WORD

In this book, we've talked about many different keys to regenerative medicine from the treatment of chronic joint, muscle, and tendon pain to the treatment of erectile dysfunction and female orgasm. We learned about stem cell and growth factor treatments to combat the effects of aging and how regenerative medicine can combat diseased organs and even future health conditions. We discussed the safety, low infection rate, results, and procedures of regenerative medicine treatments.

I'll leave you with the number-one secret for achieving great results: you must become the ambassador of your own health. You've already done some of that by reading this book, but information without action is useless.

The longer you suffer from a worsening health condition, the less likely you are to achieve optimal results from stem cell therapy or growth factor treatment, but that isn't to say you won't get results.

We know this because we have treated chronic lower back pain in ninety-year-old patients with great success. But you shouldn't put off your treatment until you reach the age of ninety! Just remember that doing something is better than doing nothing.

CONTACT INFORMATION

It has been hard to cram a great deal of information into this short book, but we tried. Because each case is different, the best thing prospective patients can do is request a free telephone consultation at one of our two facilities. Both of our facilities are used to treating patients from all over the USA and the world, and they both have a great follow-up protocol. If we believe you are a potential candidate for treatment, we will likely request medical records for further review to determine which procedure we would recommend for you.

Dr. An can be reached at the Campbell Medical Clinic in Houston, Texas. https://campbellmedicalclinic.com

Tel: 832-460-6468

Drs. Olesnicky and Hashimoto can be reached at our Desert Medical Care office in La Quinta, California.

www.DesertMedicalCare.com or www.drhdro.com

Tel: 760-777-8377

We look forward to speaking with you soon.

FURTHER READING AND REFERENCE

Now that we have reached the end of this book we would like to make known to you some of the reference materials that helped to make this book possible. If you have any further questions about what you have just read, these are excellent sources to consult.

Cheung, Emilie, et al. "Complications in Reverse Total Shoulder Arthroplasty." *Journal of the American Academy of Orthopaedic Surgeons* 19, no. 7. (July 2011): 439–449.

Ferket, Bart S., et al. "Impact of total knee replacement practice: cost effectiveness analysis of data from the Osteoarthritis Initiative." *BMJ* 356. (March 2017): https://doi.org/10.1136/bmj.j1131.

Winslow, Ron. "Common Knee Surgery Is Found to Be Worthless." *The Wall Street Journal.* July 11, 2002. https://www.wsj.com/articles/SB1026331363406125480.

Goldring, M. B., and S. R. Goldring. "Articular cartilage and subchondral bone in the pathogenesis of osteoarthritis." *Annals of the New York Academy of Sciences* 1192, no. 1. (April 2010): 230–237. https://doi.org/10.1111/j.1749-6632.2009.05240.x.

Zeckser, J., et al. "Multipotent mesenchymal stem cell treatment for discogenic low back pain and disc degeneration." *Stem Cells International.* (2015): https//doi.org/10.1155/2016/3908389.

Yelin, E. "Cost of musculoskeletal diseases: impact of work disability and functional decline." *Journal of Rheumatology* 68. (December 2003): 8–11. https://www.ncbi.nlm.nih.gov/pubmed/14712615.

Oussedik, S., et al. "Treatment of articular cartilage lesions of the knee by microfracture or autologous chondrocyte implantation: a systematic review."

Arthroscopy 31, no. 4. (April 2015): 732–744. https://doi.org/10.1016/j. arthro.2014.11.023.

Brittberg M., et al. "Treatment of deep cartilage defects in the knee with autologous chondrocyte transplantation." *The New England Journal of Medicine* 331, no. 14. (1994): 889–895. https://doi.org/10.1056/NEJM199410063311401.

Niemeyer, P., et al. "Autologous chondrocyte implantation (ACI) for cartilage defects of the knee: a guideline by the working group 'Clinical Tissue Regeneration of the German Society of Orthopaedics and Trauma (DGOU)." *Knee* 23, no. 3. (June 2016): 426–435. https://doi.org/10.1016/j.knee.2016.02.001.

Duan, L., et al. "Epigenetic regulation in chondrocyte phenotype maintenance for cell-based cartilage repair." *American Journal of Translational Research* 7, no. 11. (November 2015): 2127–2140. https://www.ncbi.nlm.nih.gov/ pubmed/26807163.

Duan, L., et al. "Cytokine networking of chondrocyte dedifferentiation in vitro and its implications for cell-based cartilage therapy." *American Journal of Translational Research* 7, no. 2. (February 2015): 192–208. https://www.ncbi. nlm.nih.gov/pubmed/25901191.

Foster, N.C., et al. "Dynamic 3D culture: models of chondrogenesis and endochondral ossification." *Birth Defects Res C Embryo Today* 105, no. 1. (March 2015): 19–33. https://doi.org/10.1002/bdrc.21088.

Park, S., and G.-I. Im. "Embryonic stem cells and induced pluripotent stem cells for skeletal regeneration." *Tissue Engineering Part B* 20, no. 5. (2014): 381–391. https://doi.org/10.1089/ten.TEB.2013.0530.

Hoben, G.M., V. P. Willard, and K. A. Athanasiou. "Fibrochondrogenesis of hESCs: growth factor combinations and cocultures." *Stem Cells and Development* 18, no. 2. (2009): 283– 292. https://doi.org/10.1089/scd.2008.0024.

Toguchida, J. "Bone and stem cells. Advancement of regenerative medicine in the locomotive system using iPS cells." *Clinical Calcium* 24, no. 4. (April 2014): 587–592. https://doi.org/CliCa1404587592.

Dulak, J., et al. "Adult stem cells: hopes and hypes of regenerative medicine." *Acta Biochimica Polonica* 62, no. 3. (2015): 329–337. https://doi.org/10.18388/abp.2015_1023.

Cheng, A., T.E. Hardingham, and S.J. Kimber. "Generating cartilage repair from pluripotent stem cells." *Tissue Engineering B* 20, no. 4. (August 2014): 257–266. https://doi.org/10.1089/ten.TEB.2012.0757.

Pacini, S. "Deterministic and stochastic approaches in the clinical application of mesenchymal stromal cells (MSCs)." *Frontiers in Cell and Developmental Biology* 2, no. 50. (September 2014): https://doi.org/10.3389/fcell.2014.00050.

Dowthwaite, G.P., et al. "The surface of articular cartilage contains a progenitor cell populations." *Journal of Cell Science* 117, no. 6. (February 2004): 889–897. https://doi.org/10.1242/jcs.00912.

Chen, S., B.H. Lee, and Y. Bae. "Notch signaling in skeletal stem cells." *Calcified Tissue International* 94, no. 1. (January 2014): 68–77. https://doi.org/10.1007/s00223-013-9773-z.

Williams, R., et al. "Identification and clonal characterisation of a progenitor cell sub-population in normal human articular cartilage." *PLoS ONE* 5, no. 10. (October 2010): e13246. https://doi.org/10.1371/journal.pone.0013246.

Koelling, S., et al. "Migratory chondrogenic progenitor cells from repair tissue during the later stages of human osteoarthritis." *Cell Stem Cell* 4, no. 4. (April 2009): 324–335. https://doi.org/10.1016/j.stem.2009.01.015.

Yu, Y., et al. "Single cell sorting identifies progenitor cell population from full thickness bovine articular cartilage." *Osteoarthritis and Cartilage* 22, no. 9. (September 2014): 318–1326. https://doi.org/10.1016/j.joca.2014.07.002.

Zhou, C., et al. "Gene expression profiles reveal that chondrogenic progenitor cells and synovial cells are closely related." *Journal of Orthopaedic Research* 32, no. 8. (August 2014): 981–988. https://doi.org/10.1002/jor.22641.

McCarthy, H.E., et al. "The comparison of equine articular cartilage progenitor cells and bone marrow-derived stromal cells as potential cell sources for cartilage repair in the horse." *Veterinary Journal* 192, no. 3. (June 2012): 345–351. https://doi.org/10.1016/j.tvjl.2001.08.036.